KW-326-210

Critical Care Focus

SM02003464
26/3/03
€14.95

HNQ K
(Gai)

WITHDRAWN
CARLISLE LIBRARY
ST MARTINS SERVICES LTD.

0727914235

Critical Care Focus

1: Renal failure

EDITOR

DR HELEN F GALLEY
Lecturer in Anaesthesia and Intensive Care
University of Aberdeen

EDITORIAL BOARD

PROFESSOR NIGEL R WEBSTER
Professor of Anaesthesia and Intensive Care
University of Aberdeen

DR PAUL GP LAWLER
Clinical Director of Intensive Care
South Cleveland Hospital

DR NEIL SONI
Consultant in Anaesthesia and Intensive Care
Chelsea and Westminster Hospital

DR MERVYN SINGER
Reader in Intensive Care
University College Hospital, London

© BMJ Books 1999
BMJ Books is an imprint of the BMJ Publishing Group

All rights reserved. No part of this publication may be reproduced, stored
in a retrieval system, or transmitted, in any form or by any means, electronic,
mechanical, photocopying, recording and/or otherwise, without the prior
written permission of the publishers.

First published in 1999
Reprinted 1999
by BMJ Books, BMA House, Tavistock Square,
London WC1H 9JR

British Library Cataloguing in Publication Data

A catalogue record for this book is available
from the British Library

ISBN 0-7279-1423-5

The chapters in this book are based on talks given at the
Intensive Care Society's 'Renal Focus Meeting', Royal Society of
Medicine, London, November 1998.

Typeset, printed and bound in Great Britain by
Latimer Trend & Company Ltd, Plymouth

Contents

Contributors

Samuel N Heyman
Hadassah University Hospital, Israel

Steve G Holt
Specialist Registrar in Anaesthesia, Royal Free Hospital, London, UK

Didier Payen
Hôpital Lariboisiere, Paris, France

William D Plant
Consultant Renal Physician, Royal Infirmary of Edinburgh, UK

Alasdair Short
Clinical Director of Intensive Care, Broomfield Hospital, Chelmsford, UK

Adrian J Voets
Department of Intensive Care, Schieland Zeikenhuis, The Netherlands

Robin G Woolfson
Consultant Renal Physician, University College, London, UK

1: Pathophysiology of acute renal failure

WILLIAM D PLANT

Clinical experience of acute renal failure

Acute renal failure (ARF) represents the abrupt collapse of many aspects of normal kidney function, in response to a complex series of insults. These frequently occur either simultaneously or in series. The complexity of this scenario is particularly apparent in already critically ill patients on the Intensive Care Unit (ICU). Unlike in the experimental situation, acute renal failure in clinical practice is an extremely "messy" pathophysiological event. Management to date remains primarily reactive. Supportive measures aim to keep the patient alive whilst/until renal function recovers.

The Madrid Acute Renal Failure Study[1] (a prospective multicentre community-based study on the epidemiology of ARF) indicates that about 200 (95% Cl 195 to 223) patients per million population (pmp) develop severe acute renal failure each year. About 1/3 (66 pmp, 95% Cl 45 to 95) of these require ICU care. Recent recommendations[2] proposed by the Renal Association and the Intensive Care Society suggest that approximately 90% of renal replacement therapy-requiring patients with isolated ARF should survive to hospital discharge. However, no more than 45–50% of patients with severe combined acute renal and respiratory failure (SCARRF), and only 5–15% of patients with multiorgan failure (MOF), as often seen in ICU, will survive (Figure 1.1).

Pathophysiological mechanisms

The underlying pathophysiology of ARF is complex, and much of the data on this has come from a variety of animal and cell culture models. The relevance of these findings to human ARF has not been extensively investigated. However, these experimental data do provide the basis of our understanding of ARF and are important starting points for the

1

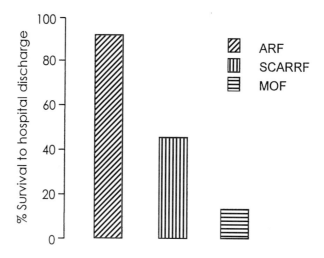

Figure 1.1   The percentage of patients requiring renal replacement therapy, those with severe combined acute renal and respiratory failure (SCARRF), those with multiorgan failure (MOF), who survive to hospital discharge.[2]

development of hypotheses and, hopefully, future novel therapeutic targets in man.

Research experience using animal models is open to question and criticism. Animal models of ARF usually vary little in genetic terms. Cell lines are, by definition, genetically identical and are designed to always respond to stimuli in a predictable and consistent manner. Experimental models therefore provide a "clean" situation quite unlike that seen clinically. As a consequence, scepticism is to be encouraged when one comes across yet another literature claim of "an exciting new breakthrough" with major potential to improve the management of human ARF. Despite these limitations, there is much to be learned from experimental renal failure. Some mechanisms are likely to occur reasonably consistently and allow formulation of a conceptual basis as to possible mechanisms of ARF in man.

Within the kidney, *cellular responses* to injury vary even in response to similar stimuli. It is perhaps helpful to view the cellular response in ARF as going through three distinct phases: initiation, maintenance and eventually recovery. Cells initially go through a phase of adaptation which may then be followed by a phase of maladaptation prior to recovery. These phases thus reflect a continuum of adaptive, maladaptive and restorative responses of tubular epithelial and vascular endothelial cells to ischaemic and toxic insults. These cells respond to injury in a variety of ways, which are further modified by the presence of a variety of mediators.

Two types of cells are critical to the initiation, maintenance and recovery phases of ARF. These are *tubular epithelial cells* and *vascular endothelial cells*.

Tubular epithelial cell damage

Despite the term "acute tubular necrosis", microscopic examination of renal biopsy specimens from patients with ARF usually reveals little histological damage. The damage is focal and localised only to certain areas of the nephron. There is often disparity between the histological appearance of a damaged kidney with acute renal failure and the level of dysfunction. When the proximal tubule is exposed, either to an ischaemic or a toxic insult, then one particular area, the straight (S3) segment, exhibits most of the histological damage. This increased susceptibility to injury probably reflects the relative hypoxia of the inner cortical/outer medullary milieu in which these segments lie. The S1 and the S2 segments are much less severely damaged. The ascending loop of Henlé, which was previously thought to be a major site of injury, is now known not to be severely affected apart from in experimental models utilising a red blood cell-free perfusate solution. Injury to the cortical collecting duct following an ischaemic or toxic insult is relatively rare.

S3 cells exposed to either an ischaemic or toxic injury respond in one of three ways. If the injury is sufficiently severe then the result is lethal and the cells will die. Classically, cell death in this situation was thought to be due to necrosis, but increasing evidence has shown the involvement of apoptotic or programmed cell death. Necrosis is a chaotic, unregulated process commonly resulting from more severe insults. Rapid depletion of intracellular energy sources and rapid destruction of the lipid bilayers of the cell membrane causes the cells to swell and eventually release their cytosolic contents into the interstitial space inducing local inflammation.

Apoptosis, however, is a genetically regulated and energy-requiring process with no inflammatory response. Apoptotic cells are cleanly and effectively removed by phagocytes. As a consequence, in acute renal failure it is very uncommon to see apoptotic cells, and other techniques are necessary to identify its presence. In many cases, although large numbers of injured renal tubular cells do die, only a few become necrotic with local inflammation. Many cells however will have also been lost through apoptosis. Thus, loss of cells may be greater than is apparent from the amount of necrosis visible on a biopsy specimen. If the initial insult is less severe, then cells may die predominantly from apoptosis rather than necrosis, particularly if sufficient energy stores are available. This can be demonstrated experimentally using the drug cisplatin, which causes tubular cell necrosis at high concentrations and apoptosis at lower concentrations.[3]

Apoptosis is genetically controlled. Cells are pre-programmed to die by apoptosis, but are often prevented from entering this cycle by exposure to so-called "survival factors". These include protein mediators, cell-to-cell adhesion molecules and other soluble factors which regulate the expression of the apoptotic processes. Thus, injured cells can, in theory, be prevented

3

from becoming apoptotic through modification of the signals which regulate apoptosis. Loss of cell adherence both to other cells and to the basement membrane are important signals for apoptotic changes.

Cells can become dysfunctional through sublethal injury. It is not so easy to determine the mechanism of loss of function when cells do not actually die, but it has been suggested that disruption of the actin cytoskeleton (which can be "seen" as loss of the brush border) may be important. There are important consequences of disruption of the cytoskeleton. Normal cell polarity, normal cell-to-cell adhesion and cell-to-basement membrane adhesion are lost. When the latter occurs then abnormal surface expression of β-1 integrins (normally confined to the basolateral aspect of the cell) may occur. The actin cytoskeleton keeps the cell in the right shape, facilitating cell-to-cell adhesion and therefore integrity of the epithelial monolayer, keeping filtrate and circulating blood separate. Tight junctions are maintained allowing paracellular movement of solutes and water and the cell is bound to its basement membrane. If the cell is sublethally injured and the actin cytoskeleton becomes disrupted then, in extreme cases, the cell may stop adhering to its neighbouring cell and simply fall off the basement membrane. The ensuing gap means that solutes and water will "flow back" (back-filtration) into the interstitium, thereby compromising renal function. Furthermore, loss of cell adhesion is an important initiating signal for apoptosis.

Loss of the actin cytoskeleton (Table 1.1) alters epithelial cell polarity and may result in the translocation of the basolateral sodium potassium ATP-ase from the basolateral aspect to the tubular surface of the cell. It may, therefore, pump sodium *into* the cell instead of *out* of it, leading to cell swelling and further dysfunction. In ARF there is frequently obstruction in the tubular lumen, often with the detritus of necrotic cells which have been lost through lethal injury. In addition, living epithelial cells which have been shed may also cause obstruction, with abnormally expressed β-1 integrins allowing cell-to-cell adhesion, aggregation of cells and resulting in raised glomerular pressure.

In summary, tubular cell damage in ARF can result from necrosis and/or apoptosis as a result of lethal injury, but perhaps more important are the changes seen as a result of sublethal insults. This typically results in damage to the actin cytoskeleton with loss of polarity and disruption of adhesion

Table 1.1 Factors in sublethal injury: consequences of disruption of the actin skeleton

- Loss of normal cell polarity
- Loss of cell-to-cell adhesion
- Loss of cell-to-basement membrane adhesion
- Abnormal expression of β-1 integrins

between cells and matrix, disruption of normal epithelial adhesion, with loss of barrier functions and shedding of cells into the lumen. The consequences include back leak of solute and water from the filtrate into the interstitium and peritubular venous system, obstruction of the tubular lumen, raised intratubular pressure and decreased glomerular filtration rate. Obstruction is typically due to proteinaceous casts which may include aggregates of tubular epithelial cells.

Endothelium effects and renal blood flow

Marked haemodynamic changes occur in acute renal failure, with reduced renal blood flow of the order of 40–50% of normal (Table 1.2). Renal blood flow varies within different regions of the kidney, which is very important for a number of reasons. Firstly, the outer medulla is relatively hypoxic, even in healthy individuals. The normal PO_2 in the outer medulla is between 5–10 mmHg, compared to about 50 mmHg in the cortex. Renal blood flow is diminished as a consequence of capillary congestion with leucocytes, platelets and red blood cells, and of intrarenal vasoconstriction, primarily due to imbalance between the actions of endothelin and nitric oxide (Table 1.3).

Exposure to an inflammatory insult (such as sepsis) or an ischaemic insult results in the release of protein mediators which promote leucocyte adhesion to vascular endothelial cells, leading to pronounced damage to the endothelium. Animal studies have shown an important role for a cell adhesion molecule (ICAM-1) in this process. Transgenic mice lacking

Table 1.2   Mechanisms affecting renal blood flow

Medullary congestion	Intrarenal vasoconstriction
Physical obstruction	*Imbalance*
leucocytes	endothelin
platelets	nitric oxide
erythrocytes	

Table 1.3   Differential physiological effects of endothelin and nitric oxide

Endothelin	Nitric oxide
Regulates nitric oxide release	Regulates endothelin release
Potent, long acting	Effects on vasculature
Local production and action	Effects on tubules
Endothelin A receptor	Nitric oxide synthase
vascular smooth muscle	type III or endothelial constitutive NOS
Endothelin B receptor	Nitric oxide synthase
vascular endothelium	type II or inducible NOS

the ICAM-1 gene do not develop acute renal failure after an ischaemic insult,[4] unlike mice who do express the ICAM-1 gene, suggesting a role for the binding of leucocytes to the endothelium in pathogenesis of ARF in response to ischaemia.

The balance between endothelium-derived nitric oxide and endothelin production also has profound effects on renal blood flow. There are three endothelin (ET) proteins – ET1, ET2 and ET3 – all of which are generated in the kidney. ET1 is the more important with regard to local renal effects. Endothelin is an extremely potent and long acting vasoconstricting agent, with both local intrarenal production and intrarenal action. It reduces renal blood flow more potently than that of any other vascular beds and, when unopposed by vasodilatory stimuli, sustains medullary vasoconstriction. Endothelin acts on two receptors. ETA receptors are predominantly located on vascular smooth muscle cells and ETB receptors on vascular endothelial cells (although this distribution exhibits considerable inter-species variation). Release of endothelin regulates nitric oxide release, thus maintaining the balance of vasoconstriction and vasodilatation.

Animal studies have shown profound species differences in the function of the endothelin receptors. In the rat the ETA receptor is responsible for vasoconstriction whilst the ETB receptor mediates its impact on nitric oxide release.[5] However, in mice, both ETA and ETB receptors mediate intrarenal vasoconstriction.[6] In man the exact function of the receptors remains unknown, although there are relatively more ETB than ETA receptors in the kidney. In sublethal injury, increased expression of the ET1 gene occurs with, in turn, increased expression of ETA receptors.

Nitric oxide is produced from L-arginine by the action of nitric oxide synthase (NOS). There are currently known to be three distinct isoforms: neuronal NOS (nNOS), also known as type I NOS; inducible NOS (iNOS), or type II NOS; and endothelial constitutive NOS (ecNOS), or type III NOS. Type III NOS activity and hence vasodilator tone, is decreased in acute renal failure, allowing vasoconstrictive forces to predominate. However, type II NOS activity is induced as part of the inflammatory response, leading to tubular cell damage as a result of local cytotoxicity. This is important because administration of nitric oxide could decrease renal vasoconstriction (direct vasodilatory effect and down-regulation of endothelin release), but may also result in increased tubular damage as it renders these cells more prone to injury.

Recovery of tubular integrity

Recovery from acute renal failure to normal structure and function requires that normally non-replicating renal tubular cells regenerate. At the onset of acute renal failure, renal tubular cells will start to express the early response genes, c-fos and egr-1.[3] Curiously, almost all of this occurs in the thick ascending loop of Henlé. The WT1 gene controls differentiation into distinct renal structures during embryonic development[7] and is not normally seen again except when the kidney is recovering from acute tubular necrosis. Growth factors may be important and cell culture studies suggest that EGF and IGF1 receptors are expressed early in acute renal failure.

In summary, disturbances in intrarenal haemodynamics, especially in medullary regional blood flow, are consistently found in ARF. Total renal blood flow is typically reduced by at least 50%, due to physical congestion or vasoconstriction. ICAM-1 mediated adhesion of leucocytes to endothelial cells may be of importance and commonly follows exposure to inflammatory mediators. The balance between vasoconstriction (endothelin 1) and vasodilatation (nitric oxide) promotes vasoconstriction. Constitutive nitric oxide release is decreased but paradoxically, and particularly in sepsis, inducible nitric oxide synthase activity may increase, leading to cytotoxic effects.

References

1 Liano F, Pascual J, The Madrid Acute Renal Failure Study Group. Epidemiology of acute renal failure: A prospective, multicentre, community-based study. *Kidney Internat* 1996;**50**:811–18.
2 The Standards and Audit Subcommittee of the Renal Association on behalf of the Renal Association and the Royal College of Physicians. *Treatment of adult patients with renal failure: recommended standards and audit measures*, 2nd Edition. *J Royal Coll Physicians Lond.* 1995;**29**:190–1.
3 Lieberthal W. Biology of acute renal failure; therapeutic implications. *Kidney Internat* 1997;**52**:1102–15.
4 Kelly K, Williams W, Colvin R, Meehan S, Springer T, Guttierrez-Ramos J-C, Bonventre J. Intercellular adhesion molecule-1-deficient mice are protected against ischaemic renal injury. *J Clin Invest* 1996;**97**:1056–63.
5 Matsura T, Miura K, Ebara T, Yukimura T, Yamanaka S, Kim S, Iwao H. Renal vascular effects of the selective endothelin receptor antagonists in anaesthetised rats. *Br J Pharmacol* 1997;**122**:81–6.
6 Berthiaume I, Yanagisawa M, Yanagisawa H, deWit D, D'Orleans-Just P. Pharmacology of endothelins in vascular circuits of normal or heterozygous endothelin-A or endothelin-B knockout transgenic mice. *J Cardiovasc Pharmacol* 1998;**31**(Suppl):S561–4.
7 Dressler GR. Transcription factors in renal development: the WT-1 and pax-s story. *Semin Nephrol* 1995;**15**:263–271.

Recommended reading

Bonventre J. Mechanisms of ischemic acute renal failure. *Kidney Internat* 1993;**43**:1160–78.
Brezis M, Rosen S. Hypoxia of the renal medulla – its implications for disease. *N Engl J Med* 1995;**332**:647–55.

2: Pressure, flow and fluid loading

ALASDAIR SHORT

The formation of glomerular filtrate is entirely dependent upon the renal perfusion pressure generated within the systemic circulation. Without a satisfactory cardiac output and perfusion pressure renal function will be impaired.

Determinants of renal blood flow

Renal blood flow is equal to the input (renal arterial) pressure minus the output (venous) pressure, divided by the resistance of the renal vascular bed. There is a critical closing pressure at which renal artery perfusion stops, estimated to be 20–30 mmHg. Increasing intra-abdominal pressure will affect renal blood flow, since venous pressure will increase as intra-abdominal pressure rises, reducing perfusion pressure. Patients with intra-abdominal pressures >25 cm H_2O will become oliguric but recover renal function when the excessive pressure is reduced, provided no other cause for renal failure is present.

Renal blood flow is about 20% of the cardiac output, approximately 400 ml/100 g per minute. The kidney is one of the most highly perfused tissues in the body in terms of blood flow per unit mass. Urine production of 1 ml per minute arises from renal blood flow of 1 litre per minute. Oxygen consumption during the process of urine production is approximately 10% of the basal VO_2 i.e. oxygen extraction is very low across the whole organ although within the outer medulla where sodium reabsorption occurs, oxygen extraction is very high. Schlichtig and co-workers[1] investigated the relationship of renal perfusion, oxygen consumption and blood flow in a dog model when oxygen delivery was reduced by haemorrhage. They demonstrated that renal oxygen consumption differs from other organs as blood flow falls. In the kidney, oxygen consumption falls in parallel with the decrease in renal blood flow, compared with the maintenance of oxygen consumption as blood flow falls to a critical point by increased oxygen extraction in other organs. When blood flow is reduced to the kidney the vasculature supplying outer cortex glomeruli shuts down first. Perfusion to the juxtamedullary glomeruli is maintained until there is complete loss of perfusion.

Renal vasculature

Within the kidney the arterioles have different muscular structures depending on whether they are within the outer cortex or the juxtamedullary area. The renal vessels are sensitive to neurohumoral agents with myogenic vessel responses to changes in intraluminal pressure mediated via calcium channels. Dilator responses to increased flow and sheer stress are mediated both by nitric oxide and prostaglandin production. The afferent arteriole appears to be tonically under the control of nitric oxide (NO). When NO synthesis is blocked, significant changes in the resistance of the afferent arteriole occur with little effect upon the efferent arteriole.

Autoregulation

Glomerular filtration rate (GFR) is maintained through autoregulation controlled by the myogenic responses of the smooth muscle cells in the afferent and efferent arterioles. The juxtaglomerular apparatus modulates glomerular haemodynamics by controlling the response of the afferent and efferent arterioles to local hormone release (e.g. angiotensin II), myogenic responses, autonomic nerve input and tubuloglomerular feedback. This system preserves GFR in the face of falling renal blood flow. The decrease in the outer cortical glomerular flow with the maintenance of juxtamedullary glomerular flow preserves the perfusion of the tubule cells, particularly in those areas of the outer medulla which normally operate at a very low oxygen tension (15–20 mmHg).

Tubuloglomerular feedback

Single nephron GFR is modulated by the quantity of sodium and chloride delivered to the distal nephron.[2] As the amount of sodium arriving at the macula densa increases (e.g. as a result of impaired proximal sodium reabsorption), single nephron GFR reduces under the influence of angiotensin II release. Sodium loading will attenuate this response although not completely block it and possibly protect the outer medulla from further hypoxic stress in the face of hypovolaemia or nephrotoxic insult. Nitric oxide is thought to play a major role in tubuloglomerular feedback.

Response to volume depletion

The response to volume depletion is initially afferent vasodilatation, with subsequent efferent vasoconstriction in an attempt to maintain enough

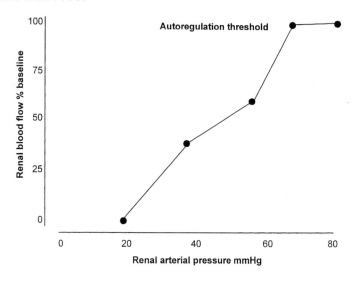

Figure 2.1 The effect of renal arterial pressure on renal blood flow demonstrating autoregulation in an awake sheep model (modified from Bersten AD, Holt AW, New Horizons *1995;3:650–61, with permission).*

pressure to continue to produce glomerular filtrate as renal blood flow decreases. Reduction in cortical filtration occurs early, with maintenance of juxtamedullary glomerular filtration. The outer medullary blood flow is maintained by the production of adenosine, prostaglandins and NO. Using an awake chronically instrumented sheep model the autoregulation threshold has been investigated.[3] The autoregulation threshold was found to be 60–80 mmHg (Figure 2.1). Indirect evidence from humans suggests a similar figure in patients who are not chronically hypertensive.[4]

Vascular injury

The renal vasculature may be injured by direct vascular injury, for example sudden systemic vascular collapse will cause ischaemia with loss of endothelium mediated vasodilatation, release of endothelin and other vasoconstrictors plus an increase in vascular permeability. Animal models of acute renal failure suggest that there is increased basal microvascular tone caused by an intrinsic vascular effect with altered vascular response to angiotensin and other constricting and dilating agents.

Acute renal failure in the Intensive Care Unit

The insults likely to impair autoregulation include prolonged haemorrhagic shock, sepsis and low cardiac output states such as myocardial pump failure and hypovolaemia. Using a rat model of acute renal failure induced by administration of noradrenaline into the renal artery, Kelleher et al.[5] showed that there was a loss of normal autoregulatory control which persisted for 1 week and had partly returned by three weeks. The renal vasculature was abnormally unresponsive to angiotensin II or noradrenaline at 1 week post insult. A similar study using a renal arterial occlusion acute renal failure model in dogs showed severe autoregulatory impairment and loss of response to changes in blood flow. A paradoxical increase in renal vascular resistance was found as blood flow fell.[6]

Prevention of acute renal failure

Inadequacy of perfusion will produce hypoxia within the outer medulla such that the kidney is vulnerable to further insults. Providing that cardiac function is adequate sodium loading will maintain cardiac output and perfusion pressure, reducing sodium reabsorption and medullary oxygen demand. In theory, renal function may be less vulnerable if oxygen consumption is reduced within the medulla of the kidney by the use of a diuretic such as furosemide. Although there have been some studies using diuretic to prevent acute renal failure there is little evidence of benefit. Patients at high risk of developing acute renal failure when given radiocontrast media are one example where diuretic prophylaxis has been studied. In animal studies there is evidence that administration of a diuretic (furosemide) plus saline would protect against radiocontrast induced acute renal failure.[7] However there is no clinical study that has demonstrated any benefit over saline loading for any loop diuretic or mannitol.[8] On the contrary the evidence suggests that diuretics adversely affect renal function when used to prevent radiocontrast nephropathy.[9] Treatment of established acute renal failure with diuretics (torosamide or furosemide) plus dopamine provided no benefit compared to saline loading alone in a randomised controlled trial,[10] despite the theoretical advantages of decreased tubular oxygen consumption and wash out of tubular debris causing obstruction. Excessive diuresis may lead to volume depletion and aggressive cardiovascular support and sodium loading seems to be at least as good as diuretic treatment.

Maintenance of an effective circulating volume and an adequate cardiac output with restoration of perfusion pressure to 80 mmHg (or higher in previously hypertensive patients) has been recommended. Dobutamine therapy has been compared to dopamine in a randomised trial in the Intensive Care Unit and found to provide better outcome for renal function.[11] When peripheral vascular resistance is low, evidence supports the use of a vasoconstrictor such as noradrenaline (nonepinephrine).[12–15]

In an attempt to prevent the development of established renal failure, we have adopted in patients with meningococcal septicaemia, an early

11

treatment protocol, which includes antibiotics, sodium loading with central venous pressure control and noradrenaline (nonepinephrine) to support mean arterial pressure as soon as the patient presents to hospital. This treatment is initiated in the Accident and Emergency Department. The following two recent cases describe what may be achieved. The first was a 19-year-old previously fit man who had been unwell for 24 hours. His mean arterial pressure was 68 mmHg and he had a base deficit of −12. He was thrombocytopenic and his serum creatinine was 200 μmol/l. His urine output was negligible for the first hour. He was volume loaded until his CVP increased and then noradrenaline was started. Over the next few hours diuresis was satisfactory and weaning from noradrenaline was commenced as his mean arterial pressure began to return to normal over the next 48–72 hours. The second case was a young woman of 17 who was admitted to the Accident and Emergency Department in a confused, hypotensive state, with a mean arterial pressure of 55 mmHg. She was severely oliguric and her serum creatinine was 250 μmol/l, with a base deficit of −10. After only three days renal function had improved following volume expansion and noradrenaline with maintenance of perfusion pressure. The response to noradrenaline and change in serum creatinine in these two patients are shown in Figures 2.2 and 2.3 respectively. It is impossible from two case reports to prove that this regime alone prevented the further development of acute renal failure but it illustrates the principles that have been shown to be of importance.

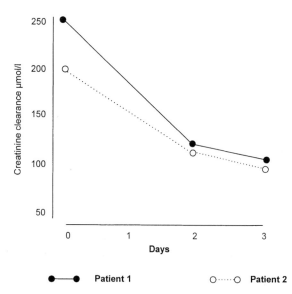

Figure 2.2   The response of mean arterial pressure and urine volume to an early treatment protocol, which includes antibiotics, sodium loading with central venous pressure control and noradrenaline initiated in the Accident and Emergency Department, in a 19-year-old man (see text for full details).

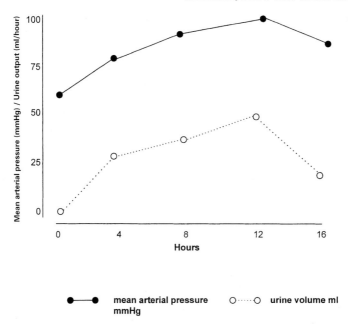

Figure 2.3   The response of creatinine clearance to an early treatment protocol, which includes antibiotics, sodium loading with central venous pressure control and noradrenaline initiated in the Accident and Emergency Department, in two patients (see text for full details).

Summary

It has been difficult to reproduce in animals the typical sequence of multiple insults to renal function that frequently occur in patients. Commonly patients are hypotensive, with severe vascular disease, cardiac failure, sepsis and are receiving nephrotoxic drugs. It seems that there is no magical treatment likely to be available for the foreseeable future to reverse acute renal failure. Until then, the goals should be to restore effective circulating volume, ensure adequate cardiac output and adequate perfusion pressure.

References

1 Schlichtig R, Kramer DJ, Boston JR, Pinsky MR. Renal oxygen consumption during progressive hemorrhage. *J Applied Physiol* 1991;**70**:1957–62.
2 Ito S, Carretero OA, Abe K. Nitric oxide in the regulation of renal blood flow. *New Horizons* 1995;**3**:615–23.
3 Bersten AD, Holt AW. Vasoactive drugs and the importance of renal perfusion pressure. *New Horizons* 1995;**3**:650–61.
4 Stone AM and Stahl WM, Renal effects of hemorrhage in normal men. *Ann Surg* 1970;**172**:825–36.

5 Kelleher SP, Robinette JB, and Conger JD. Sympathetic nervous system in the loss of autoregulation in accute renal failure. *Am J of Physiol* 1984;**246**:F379–86.

6 Adams PL, Adams FF, Bell PD and Navar LG. Impaired renal blood flow autoregulation in accute renal failure. *Kidney Internat* 1980;**18**:68–76.

7 Heyman SN, Brezis M, Greenfield Z, Rosen S. Protective role of furosemide and saline in radiocontrast-induced renal failure in the rat. *Am J Kidney Dis* 1989;**14**:377–85.

8 Solomon R, Werner C, Mann D, D'Elia J, Silva P. Effects of saline, mannitol, and furosemide to prevent acute decreases in renal function induced by radiocontrast agents. *N Engl J Med* 1994;**331**:1416–20.

9 Weinstein JM, Heyman S, Brezis M. Potential deleterious effect of furosemide in radiocontrast nephropathy. *Nephron* 1992;**62**:413–15.

10 Shilliday IR, Quinn JK, Allison ME. Loop diuretics in the management of acute renal failure: a prospective, double blind, placebo controlled, randomized study. *Nephrol Dial Transplant* 1997;**12**:2592–6.

11 Duke GJ, Briedis JH, Weaver RA. Renal support in critically ill patients: low dose dopamine or low dose dobutamine. *Crit Care Med* 1994;**22**:1919–25.

12 Desjars P, Pinaud M, Potel G, Tasseau F, Touze MD. A reappraisal of norepinephrine therapy in human septic shock. *Crit Care Med* 1987;**15**:134–7.

13 Hesselvik JF, Brodin B. Low dose norepinephrine in patients with septic shock and oliguria: effects on afterload, urine flow and oxygene transport. *Crit Care Med* 1989;**17**:179–80.

14 Marin C, Eon B, Saux P, Aknin P, Gouin F. Renal effects of norepinephrine used to treat septic shock patients. *Crit Care Med* 1990;**18**:282–5.

15 Redl-Wenzl EM, Armbruster C, Edelmann G, *et al.* The effects of norepinephrine on hemodynamics and renal function in septic shock states. *Intensive Care Med* 1993;**19**:151–4.

3: Rhabdomyolysis

STEVE G HOLT

What is rhabdomyolysis?

Rhabdomyolysis occurs when there is massive breakdown of muscle with release of myocyte contents into the circulation, often following trauma. The pathology of myocyte cell death shares a final common pathway involving an increase in intracytoplasmic calcium. While muscle breakdown may not in itself be life threatening, the toxic cocktail released into the circulation may cause profound metabolic upset and secondary organ dysfunction, particularly since muscle makes up 40% of total body mass. The kidney often takes the brunt of this metabolic derangement and its exposure to toxic myoglobin species results in acute renal failure in a proportion of cases. Treatment has been directed at renoprotective strategies and advances in our understanding of the pathophysiology of the acute renal failure are likely to result in improved treatment regimes in the next few years. Prediction of those patients with biochemical evidence of muscle damage (raised creatine kinase) who are at risk of developing acute renal failure remains difficult, although a scoring system has been developed predicting a 50% chance of developing acute renal failure (Table 3.1).

Rhabdomyolysis is an important cause of acute renal failure. The first suggestion of a link between rhabdomyolysis and acute renal failure came during the Second World War when the association of brown pigment casts and crush injury was noted. These casts were later shown to be myoglobin and probably the toxic insult to the kidney. Between 17–40%

Table 3.1 "Ward score".[1] Predictive factors identified for developing ARF. A score of 7 or more implies a >50% incidence of ARF on regression analysis.

Points	−4	−3	−2	−1	0	1	2	3	4	5	6	7	8	9	10
PO_4^{2-}					0.65	0.97	1.29	1.61	1.94	2.26	2.58	2.91	3.23	3.55	
K^+							2.5	3.1	3.7	4.4	5	5.6	6.2	6.8	7.4
Albumin		46	35	23											
CK >6,000					No	Yes									
Dehydration					No		Yes								
Sepsis					No		Yes								

of patients with rhabdomyolysis go on to develop acute renal failure, and rhabdomyolysis accounts for 8–15% of all cases of acute renal failure in the United States.

Mechanisms of acute renal failure in rhabdomyolysis

The mechanism for the ARF of rhabdomyolysis has been extensively studied but we have only recently begun to understand the pathophysiology of this condition. There are a number of pathways through which the released myocyte debris can be nephrotoxic.

Tubular obstruction

Myoglobin has a molecular weight of about 17 KDa and is therefore easily filtered and deposited in the kidney tubules. This can be seen microscopically as dark brown staining in the tubules of animals given glycerol, which provides a good model of rhabdomyolysis. The presence of anionic Tamm-Horsfall protein in the urine decreases the solubility of myoglobin and combines to form the so-called "brown sugar casts", visible microscopically. In addition, increased urate load from myocyte breakdown can precipitate in the urine, contributing to obstruction. However, micropuncture experiments show that intratubular pressures are normal and there is no tubular back-leak,[2] suggesting that tubular obstruction is not the most important cause of acute renal failure. A reduction in urinary pH increases the solubility of myoglobin in urine due to effects on Tamm-Horsfall protein, but this does not necessarily reduce the total myoglobin burden on the kidney.

Tubular necrosis

Tubular necrosis can occur throughout the nephron and there is accumulating evidence that free radical injury is involved. Free radical mediated injury can affect many parts of the cell including lipids, DNA and protein, and has been implicated in the pathogenesis of cellular dysfunction in a number of conditions. There is both induction and consumption of antioxidant enzymes in rhabdomyolysis. Previously thiobarbituric acid reactive substances have been measured and shown to be elevated, indicative of lipid peroxidation. However methodological problems exist in the measurement of these substances with *ex vivo* artefactal generation. Recently a group of lipid peroxides, the F_2-isoprostanes have been discovered. These are prostaglandin-like molecules which are produced by the action of free radicals on arachidonic acid present in cell membranes and other lipids. Esterified isoprostanes formed in this way can be measured within tissues localising lipid peroxidation. Isoprostanes are then cleaved by a

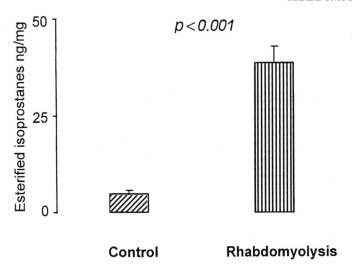

Figure 3.1   Esterified isoprostanes found in kidneys of animals injected i.m. with glycerol, indicating enhanced lipid peroxidation (modified from Moore et al.[4] 1998).

phospholipase and can then be measured as free isoprostanes in the plasma and in urine, and this has now been well validated as a model for *in vitro* and *in vivo* lipid peroxidation, reflecting oxidant injury. Isoprostanes can be measured by gas chromatography mass spectrometry (GCMS) and immunoassay kits are also now available.

Previous studies have implicated "free" iron, released from myoglobin, in the mechanism of free radical generation by Fenton chemistry in the kidney in acute renal failure due to rhabdomyolysis.[3] However, we have shown that even in the presence of iron chelating agents, myoglobin can cause oxidative injury and lipid peroxidation, effectively excluding a mechanism for "free" iron. In animal models of rhabdomyolysis we have localised lipid peroxidation to kidney, as shown by increased esterified isoprostanes (Figure 3.1).

Iron in myoglobin is normally present in the ferrous (Fe^{2+}) state in muscle and is incapable of causing lipid peroxidation alone. When deposited in the kidney it oxidises to the ferric (Fe^{3+}) state. Redox cycling between the ferric and ferryl (Fe^{4+}) states can then occur causing lipid peroxidation and renal damage. This reaction can be initiated by lipids themselves, unlike Fenton chemistry where free iron requires hydroxyl radicals to cause lipid peroxidation.[4]

Reduction in renal blood flow

Renal vasoconstriction can occur, due in part to homeostatic mechanisms associated with blood and fluid losses from a traumatic injury. Infusion of myoglobin itself can cause vasoconstriction and other mediators have been implicated, including endothelin, nitric oxide, thromboxane and isoprostanes. In addition there is evidence of up-regulation of inflammatory mediators including tumour necrosis factor α. It is interesting to note that intravenous infusions of very small concentrations of isoprostanes raise the blood pressure and reduce renal blood flow. Infusion into the renal artery almost completely shuts off blood flow to the kidney, by acting on thromboxane A2-like receptors and possibly by causing endothelin release.

Therapeutic strategies

Early fluid resuscitation is the most important therapeutic intervention in rhabdomyolysis. Guidelines suggest intensive fluid resuscitation with the administration of 10–12 litres of fluid over 24 hours to achieve a diuresis of 200–300 ml per hour. One replacement fluid suggested consists of sodium 110 mmol/l, chloride 70 mmol/l, bicarbonate 40 mmol/l, glucose 5 g/100 ml with 10 mg/l of mannitol.[5] In an animal model of rhabdomyolysis, the fall in creatinine clearance seen after rhabdomyolysis can be partially prevented with alkalinisation (Figure 3.2). The mechanism for this effect may relate to increased myoglobin solubility and decreased tubular precipitation, but alkalinisation markedly reduces lipid peroxide formation, attenuating free radical mediated damage (Figure 3.3). This is likely to be due to increased stability of ferrylMb at pH8, compared to pH5, such that redox cycling is inhibited.

Mannitol has also been advocated but has not been shown to be better than volume diuresis alone,[4] and may even be harmful. Other antioxidants have also been used therapeutically in the prevention of renal failure in

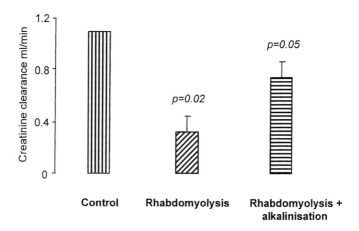

Figure 3.2   Creatinine clearance is improved by alkalinisation in the glycerol model (modified from Moore et al.[4] 1998).

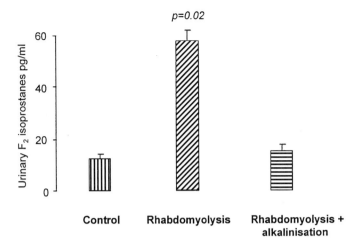

Figure 3.3   Urinary isoprostanes are suppressed by alkalinisation in the glycerol model (modified from Moore et al.[4] 1998).

experimental models including 21 aminosteroids, 2,3 dihydrobenzoate and dimethylurea.

There are a few anecdotal reports of the use of extracorporeal circuits to remove myoglobin and thereby reduce the burden on the kidney. Myoglobin can certainly be removed from solution by plasmapheresis, diafiltration, haemodialysis or charcoal haemoperfusion, but clinical application remains unclear given the short half life of myoglobin, and the prohibitive cost and complications of such therapy. Other therapies include thromboxane receptor and endothelin antagonists.

Summary

About 80% of people survive from the acute renal failure of rhabdomyolysis. Renal recovery is usual within 3 months, unless complicated by sepsis or other organ dysfunction. Rhabdomyolysis is a relatively common cause of acute renal failure. Prevention of renal failure depends on prompt resuscitation with fluid and alkali. The mechanism of acute renal failure is likely to involve free radical damage and therapeutic alkalisation can ameliorate this. New therapeutic approaches involving antioxidant strategies are likely to be the focus of future studies.

References

1 Ward MM. Factors predictive of acute renal failure in rhabdomyolysis. *Arch Intern Med* 1988;**148**:1553–7.

2 Oken DE, DiBona GF, McDonald FD. Micropuncture studies of the recovery phase of myohemoglobinuric acute renal failure in the rat. *J Clin Invest* 1970;**49**:730–7.
3 Zager RA, Foerder CA. Effects of inorganic iron and myoglobin on *in vitro* proximal tubular lipid peroxidation and cytotoxicity. *J Clin Invest* 1992;**89**:989–95.
4 Moore KP, Holt SG, Patel RP *et al.* A causative role for redox cycling of myoglobin and its inhibition by alkalinization in the pathogenesis and treatment of rhabdomyolysis-induced renal failure. *J Biol Chem* 1998;**273**:31731–7.
5 Better OS, Stein JH. Early management of shock and prophylaxis of acute renal failure in traumatic rhabdomyolysis *N Engl J Med* 1990;**322**:825–9.

4: Nephrotoxic compounds in the Intensive Care Unit

ALASDAIR SHORT

Nephrotoxic reactions to drugs and other compounds are relatively common and have been described for many substances, several of which are drugs commonly encountered within the Intensive Care Unit. They are commonly associated with renal dysfunction in patients in the Intensive Care Unit although the incidence of drug induced renal failure is unclear. Any estimate of incidence is complicated by the multifactorial nature of the causes of acute renal failure in the intensive care patient.

Mechanisms of nephrotoxicity

There are several mechanisms by which nephrotoxicity may arise (Table 4.1). These include general and local vascular effects, direct effects on renal tubules, tubular obstruction and acute interstitial nephritis. Acute glomerulonephritis can also occur although this is rare.

Vascular effects

Diuretics and β blockers can cause low cardiac output states and systemic vasodilating agents such as sodium nitroprusside or angiotensin converting enzyme inhibitors may reduce renal perfusion. Drugs which have a direct effect on the renal vasculature predispose to renal failure. Angiotensin has paracrine actions within the glomerular circulation. The use of angiotensin converting enzyme (ACE) inhibitors not only inhibits angiotensin production but also interferes with bradykinin which has an important role in circulatory control within the glomerulus. Non-steroidal anti-inflammatory drugs (NSAIDs) and cyclosporin A cause vasoconstriction within the renal circulation with major effects on medullary blood flow and oxygen delivery.

Direct injury to tubular cells

Proximal tubule

Several drugs have direct nephrotoxic effects on proximal tubular cells. Antibiotics (e.g. aminoglycosides and vancomycin), antifungal agents (amphotericin), and cytotoxic agents such as cisplatin are well known for their damaging action on tubular function. The damaging effects of radiocontrast media on the kidney are well recognised, and will be discussed later. Heavy metals, e.g. mercury, organic solvents such as carbon tetrahydrochloride, plant and animal toxins can also cause renal failure (Table 4.1).

Mannitol in high dosage (as well as being an osmotic diuretic) can cause proximal tubular damage as a result of excessive osmotic effects within the proximal tubule. In the oxygen-stressed environment of the outer medulla the tubule is not capable of dealing with the enormous quantity of solute that is delivered to the tubule. Tubular cells lose polarity, develop vacuoles and separate from the basement membrane. Significant electrolyte derangement may also occur due to the effects on the distal tubule affecting water reabsorption.

High dose immunoglobulin therapy may cause acute renal dysfunction by a similar process to mannitol. This was noticed after acute anuria was reported in patients on the Intensive Care Unit receiving immunoglobulin for Guillain-Barré syndrome.

Distal tubule

The actions of drugs which damage the distal tubule cause disturbance of the fine control of sodium, potassium, hydrogen ion and water balance.

Table 4.1   Mechanisms of nephrotoxicity

Mechanism of toxic effect		Nephrotoxic agent-examples
Cardiovascular		
	general	diuretics, β blockers, vasodilators
	local	ACE inhibitors, cyclosporin A
Direct tubular effect		
	proximal	aminoglycosides, amphotericin B, cisplatin, radiocontrast media, heavy metals, organic solvents, toxins, immunoglobulin, mannitol
	distal	NSAIDs, ACE inhibitors, cyclosporin A, lithium, cyclophosphamide, amphotericin B
Tubular obstruction		sulphonamides, acyclovir, tumour lysis syndrome, ethylene glycol, indinavir
Acute interstitial nephritis		β lactams, vancomycin, rifampicin, sulphonamides, ciprofloxacin, NSAID, ranitidine, cimetidine, furosemide, thiazides, phenytoin
Acute glomerulonephritis		penicillamine

Non-steroidal anti-inflammatory agents, ACE inhibitors and cyclosporin A all alter potassium balance resulting in hyperkalaemia. NSAIDs and cyclosporin A also block the compensatory mechanisms which protect blood flow to the tubule in the volume-stressed kidney.

Within the older population, approximately 1 in 1000 people are receiving lithium therapy. Chronic administration of lithium has toxic effects on distal tubular function. It causes chronic damage to the tubule with initially functional and then permanent inability to conserve water, causing nephrogenic diabetes insipidus. Acute lithium intoxication causes a similar tubular effect which may be reversible.

High dose cyclophosphamide and amphotericin B both have actions on the distal tubule which may result in hyponatraemia by impairing the kidneys' ability to excrete a water load.

Tubular obstruction

The increased use of sulphonamides in high dosage for the treatment of pneumocystis pneumonia in patients with AIDS and other immunosuppressed states has increased the incidence of crystalluria, causing tubular obstruction with renal dysfunction. This can be prevented by adequate salt and water loading to ensure adequate tubular filtrate flow to prevent precipitation of the drug. Other newer drugs have similar toxic actions e.g. the anti-viral agent acyclovir and the protease inhibitor indinavir.

Other drugs may cause uric acid crystal nephropathy as in the tumour lysis syndrome. High dose chemotherapy for haematological malignancies can result in rapid cytolytic effects resulting in a hugely increased uric acid load to the kidney. Again, unless adequate urine flow and sodium diuresis is maintained, acute crystalluria may develop. Ethylene glycol poisoning is relatively common in socially deprived areas, and as a result of its metabolism produces a large oxalate load which may crystallise in the tubule particularly as the patients are commonly volume depleted.

Acute interstitial nephritis

The commonest cause of drug induced acute interstitial nephritis is antibiotic usage, particularly the β lactams, rifampicin, sulphonamides, vancomycin and ciprofloxacin. Diuretics, including thiazides and furosemide and similarly, NSAIDs also can cause acute interstitial nephritis. Less commonly, ranitidine, cimetidine, and phenytoin cause similar damage. The mechanism for the damage is an acute allergic reaction, with infiltration of immune effector cells causing direct cytotoxicity. Nephrotoxicity increases in the presence of other predisposing factors (volume depletion, hypotension), and the decision to use a particular drug must be made taking into account the balance of risk to benefit in the individual patient's circumstances.

Acute glomerulonephritis

The development of acute glomerulonephritis is a rare complication of drugs such as penicillamine and NSAIDs.

Pre-disposing factors

Age

Although it is generally considered that age may be important in pre-disposing to renal toxicity, age *per se* is probably less important than other co-morbidities inherent in an older population. It is still unclear whether renal function significantly declines with age in the otherwise healthy elderly, although this has certainly been assumed previously. There are other more relevant factors which must be taken into consideration if nephrotoxic agents must be used.

Pre-existing renal impairment

Impaired renal function is an important factor. Nephron mass is diminished yet the kidney must continue to clear the same amount of solute per day. The load to the individual nephrons is higher. As nephron work increases, oxygen consumption increases and there is often damage to juxtamedullary glomeruli such that functional reserve is severely depleted. These patients are therefore less able to compensate for drug induced effects. There are also the problems caused by impaired drug elimination causing toxic drug levels with consequent positive feedback on the nephrotoxic process.

Sepsis

In patients with sepsis, intrinsic vascular abnormalities occur as part of the inflammatory response and pre-dispose these patients to nephrotoxicity.

Liver disease

Patients with acute or chronic hepatic disease have abnormal drug handling within the liver and commonly have abnormal intrarenal haemo-dynamics with avid salt retention which potentiates any nephrotoxicity.

Diabetes mellitus

The diabetic patient presents a particular problem. The vascular endothelium is globally abnormal in patients with diabetes. Within the kidney, the ability of the endothelium to produce endothelin or nitric oxide

Table 4.2   Factors which predipose to nephrotoxicity

- Impaired renal perfusion pressure – sodium depletion, diuretic therapy, low cardiac output
- Previously impaired renal function
- Vascular disease
- Severe infection
- Diabetes
- Liver disease

in response to stress is severely impaired, therefore limiting any defence against nephrotoxic insult.

In general there are two main categories in which the pre-disposition to renal damage is increased (Table 4.2): 1. impaired renal perfusion pressure due to sodium depletion, diuretic therapy, low cardiac output or any other condition that will promote an increased state of sodium reabsorption; 2. previously impaired renal function, vascular disease, severe infection, diabetes and liver disease.

Radiocontrast nephrotoxicity

Renal damage as a result of radiocontrast investigations is becoming so common that this cause of acute renal failure in at risk patients deserves particular mention. Radiocontrast medium in high doses is administered for CT scans and many types of vascular surgery. The major risk factors which pre-dispose to renal damage are pre-existing renal impairment, and diabetes mellitus. In the patients with both diabetes and renal dysfunction, the incidence of further renal impairment following administration of radiocontrast is over 50%. Between 1976 and 1984 a self-reporting register in the USA quantified the incidence of side effects from radiocontrast media administration. This showed the difference in the incidence of renal failure depending on whether the radiocontrast agents used was high osmolar, ionised low osmolar or non-ionised low osmolar contrast media (Figure 4.1). As time went on however the number of episodes of acute renal failure associated with the low osmolar non-ionised agents increased almost certainly as a result of the increasing amounts of contrast administered in higher risk patients

The incidence of acute renal failure after coronary interventions is consistently much higher in patients with diabetes.[1,2] Initially vasoconstriction occurs and it remains unclear whether vasoconstriction or direct tubular damage causes the damage. It has been suggested that the endothelium is particularly important within this mechanism of toxicity and in animal studies endothelin antagonists have been shown to be beneficial. Further studies in man may now be warranted. In humans to date the only preventative measure that has been proven of benefit is to ensure a saline diuresis prior to contrast administration.

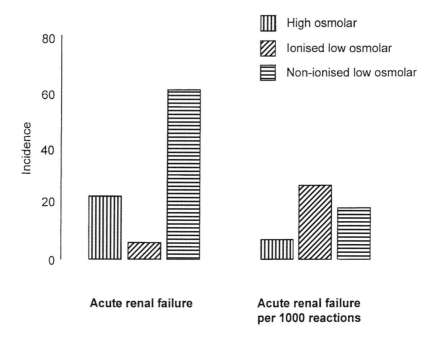

Figure 4.1   The reported incidence to the Federal Drug Authority in the USA from 1990–1994 of nephrotoxicity according to the type of radiocontrast agent used.

Within the intensive care unit contrast studies are required for vascular disease, establishing bleeding source or pancreatitis. These patients are commonly cardiovascularly unstable with pre-existing renal impairment, sepsis, diabetes and vascular disease. It is essential that meticulous care be given to ensuring adequate intravascular volume expansion and renal perfusion pressure to minimise the risk of worsening renal function.

Non-steroidal anti-inflammatory agents

Non-steroidal anti-inflammatory agents are commonly used. Their primary renal effect is inhibition of prostanoid synthesis, which therefore affects the protective maintenance of vascular perfusion and oxygen delivery within the outer medulla. These drugs selectively inhibit constitutive cyclo-oxygenase, and their effects are potentiated by hypovolaemia, low cardiac output, sepsis, liver disease and pre-existing renal failure.

Example case report

A 47-year-old man was involved in a road traffic accident and ruptured his superior gluteal artery, and sustained a fractured femur and pelvis. He required immediate operation on admission to hospital and required 25 units of blood in the perioperative period. Five days later he developed a fever but was passing urine and his renal function in terms of creatinine and urine volume was normal. His blood pressure was well maintained with a modest dose of dobutamine. He was given diclofenac for its antipyretic and analgesic properties. After a single 100 mg dose he became oliguric over the next 6 hours and his creatinine increased to the level at which renal replacement therapy was instituted and continued for a period of 3 weeks. There was no change in cardiac output or blood pressure.

This case clearly illustrates the problem of the intensive care patient administered a potentially nephrotoxic drug. The kidney is stressed due to sepsis and autoregulatory mechanisms are severely impaired because of a period of shock arising from haemorrhage. The patient was not receiving any other nephrotoxins and his blood pressure remained unchanged. Non-steroidal anti-inflammatory agents are useful drugs but may cause problems in the acutely stressed patient and in terms of prevention of nephrotoxicity, these drugs should be avoided in the Intensive Care Unit.

Prevention of nephrotoxicity

When the use of nephrotoxic agents is unavoidable, close monitoring of concentration is necessary e.g. the aminoglycosides. It is important to remember that when renal function changes pharmacokinetics alter considerably. Meticulous attention should be paid to the avoidance of hypovolaemia, reduced renal perfusion pressure and reduced cardiac output at all times, and particularly if acute nephrotoxic exposure is planned, such as radiocontrast media. No specific preventative therapies have been shown to be superior to sodium loading prior to exposure.

Summary

Maintenance of circulating volume, cardiac output and perfusion pressure to reduce stress on the kidney, and minimise medullary oxygen demand in the face of impaired oxygen delivery is recommended. Attention to the detailed management of the systemic circulation will minimise the nephrotoxic potential of potentially nephrotoxic agents that are unavoidable for proper patient management.

References

1 Weisberg LS, Kurnik PB, Kurnik BR. Risk of radiocontrast nephropathy in patients with and without diabetes mellitus. *Kidney International* 1994;**45**:259–65.
2 McCullough PA, Wolyn R, Rocher LL, Levin RN, O'Neill WW. Acute renal failure after coronary intervention: incidence, risk factors and relationship to mortality. *Am J Med* 1997;**103**:368–75.

5: Use of haemofiltration in sepsis

DIDIER PAYEN

Introduction

This review will focus not on the technical issues relating to haemofiltration as an alternative to intermittent haemodialysis for renal support, but on a view of haemofiltration as a treatment for acute inflammation or sepsis. Over the last ten years there have been some studies which have demonstrated benefit of haemofiltration in sepsis, in terms of morbidity and mortality.[1-4] All studies except for the British one published in the *Lancet* in 1994,[4] were uncontrolled with small numbers of patients and most were retrospective. In addition, the mechanisms by which such a technique may play a positive role were only suspected.

The sepsis puzzle

Figure 5.1 shows a schematic and idealised so-called sepsis puzzle, which could also be a SIRS puzzle, a trauma puzzle or an ARDS puzzle. It simply serves to illustrate the complex interaction between the components of the response to inflammation. The many studies over the last decade which targeted a single inflammatory mediator or molecule – the so-called magic bullet – revealed that this was not a good approach.[5] This was due primarily to the fact that the pro-inflammatory mediators thought to be so damaging also had a vital role in the stimulation of the production of anti-inflammatory mediators and were important for the resolution of injury. In contrast, however, haemofiltration may play a role in the regulation of both anti- and pro-inflammatory mediators, maintaining the balance[6] and hence benefiting the circulatory and metabolic consequences of acute injury. Perhaps the most important consideration for haemofiltration, is the time at which any intervention takes place.

Timing

Patients never present with a single insult, a clear cut scenario; what most often happens is a combination of trauma, haemorrhage, infection, surgery

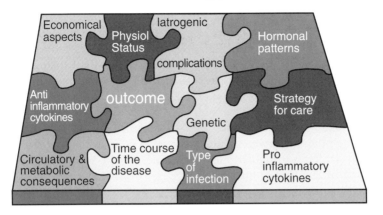

Figure 5.1   The "sepsis puzzle" showing the various factors which contribute to outcome in patients with sepsis. The same puzzle pieces could also be applied to the trauma patients, post-operative patients, those with the systemic inflammatory response syndrome (SIRS) or acute respiratory distress syndrome (ARDS).

and finally perhaps nosocomial infection. Many studies have demonstrated that even a small insult in a stressed patient will result initially in a regional or a systemic hyper-inflammatory response followed by a very rapid anti-inflammatory response. This occurs after only a few hours and is followed by immunodepression – and has been termed post-aggressive immunodepression.[7] The time point for intervention depends on the therapeutic targets, how monitoring will be performed, will effects be aimed at regional or systemic targets, and what is the benefit versus the risk?

From support to therapy

The concept of haemofiltration not as renal support but as a therapeutic intervention technique in the systemic inflammatory response may not be widely accepted, but a close look at the literature reveals the mechanisms of the mode of action of this therapy (Table 5.1). As a therapy, continuous haemofiltration should offer good tolerance and safety, adequate biocompatibility and positive interactions with the endogenous immune system. It is clear that continuous haemofiltration removes the

Table 5.1   Possible mechanisms for the beneficial effects of haemofiltration

- Fluid control
- Endotoxin – adsorption or filtration
- Cytokines – adsorption or filtration
- Cellular function – monocytes, neutrophils, lymphocytes
- Other mediators – prostaglandins, nitric oxide, endothelin

29

excess intravascular and extravascular fluid. This is important not only to reduce fluid volume, but also to control the content of this fluid and the environment of the cells which it bathes. For example cells exposed to low or high glucose levels respond differently to endotoxin.[8] In the presence of 4 mM glucose, the tumour necrosis factor α (TNFα) response of cells to endotoxin is small. If cells are exposed to 10 mM glucose, however, the TNF response is increased five fold.[9]

Interstitial fluid volume may also be reduced by haemofiltration by facilitating pumping towards the intravascular compartment and may help to optimise left ventricular filling pressures. Acid base status may be improved by the use of different buffers, for example lactate, bicarbonate or acetate.

Biocompatibility

The well monitored machines and circuits available today means that continuous haemofiltration is safe and well tolerated, acceptable to clinicians and allows excellent control of body fluid. The term biocompatibility is the ability of the filtration membrane to be tolerated by human cells, with minimum cell activation. However, there are many potential immune responses which could be used to define biocompatibility and one type of membrane may not satisfy all criteria.

Mechanisms of action of haemofiltration

Haemofiltration may affect both endogenous immune function and/or tissue tolerance of acute stress. Although the effect of body fluid control is well demonstrated and accepted, it has no real consequences in terms of improvement of organ dysfunction or in terms of outcome. Endotoxin clearing by adsorption or filtration may be beneficial, but previous studies have not categorically shown that endotoxin in the plasma is related to patient outcome. Cytokine elimination may also be a target for benefit. The majority of cytokines are too large to be filtered since membrane cut off points are approximately 30 kDa and many cytokines are larger than 30 kDa. However adsorption of cytokines to the membrane may be the mechanism by which cytokine levels can be reduced.

In the lung, haemofiltration improves gas exchange. This is related to the extravascular lung water content which is reduced by haemofiltration. Metabolic function is also improved, thus increasing clearance properties of the lung and the prostaglandin-producing capability. Cardiovascular function is also benefited – myocyte contraction is better preserved with haemofiltration but there are still no clear clinical data showing that haemofiltration is able to reduce the number and the severity of organ failures. In post-operative cardiac surgical patients, haemofiltration reduced the duration of mechanical ventilation and the length of Intensive Care Unit stay.[10,11] This was explained at least by modulation of complement activation, which was reduced in the treated group compared to the non-treated group.

Animal studies

Using a pig model of sepsis, the effect of continuous arterial venous haemofiltration on morbidity and mortality, and the inflammatory action of the ultrafiltrate, has been investigated.[12] In this severe model of sepsis (mortality 100%), animals were rendered septic by the infusion of 8×10^9 CFU S*taphylococcus aureas*. Pigs were randomised to receive either haemofiltration at different filtration rates, low, medium and fast or no filtration. It was found that survival rate was highest using membranes with the largest pore size. In a second study using a 100 kD membrane, which provides haemofiltration close to plasmaphoresis membrane size, all animals survived. In addition, injection of the ultrafiltrate into healthy animals resulted in high mortality. These results clearly suggest that haemofiltration is removing a mediator or mediators which is/are implicated in organ function during the acute phase of inflammation.

Using an *E. coli* dog model of sepsis, Gomez *et al.* demonstrated that haemofiltration was able to reverse myocardial depression.[13] Other studies have shown in endotoxin shock models that the ultrafiltrate contains factors which increase pulmonary artery pressure and depress cardiac performance in healthy animals.[14] Similar results were obtained using haemoadsorption only, i.e. no filtration. Using a non-resuscitated rabbit endotoxic shock model, mean arterial pressure was better maintained in animals treated with haemoadsorption.[15] Endotoxin clearance was more rapid in haemoadsorbed animals than controls and TNF responses were attenuated.[16] Hypocontractility of vessels was improved by haemoadsorption, with recovery of the normal contractile function of the vessel.

Using perhaps a relatively more clinically relevant model of porcine acute peritonitis following caecal ligation and puncture, the effect of continuous arteriovenous haemofiltration on the phagocytic capability of polymorphonuclear cells was assessed.[17] The study revealed that although phagocytosis of candida was lower in animals receiving filtration than controls, the phagocytic capacity of cells recovered after 72 hours.

Clinical studies

A Japanese group showed that in 16 patients with sepsis and multiorgan failure, 2 hours haemoperfusion using polymixin B fibres, which is an endotoxin chelating substance, improved hypotension in these patients.[18] Mortality was 44%, but the significance of this remains unclear, since the study was uncontrolled.

Another study showed that in 20 endotoxaemic patients, post-haemodialysis endotoxin concentrations were reduced with both poly-acrylnitril and cupraphane membranes.[19] However, with regard to removal of cytokines, one must consider the concept of the tip of the iceberg, first proposed by Cavaillon.[20] In order for the circulating plasma levels to increase, both origin cells and target cells must be saturated for concentrations to increase in the extracellular fluid. Thus removal of cytokines from the plasma may have little effect in terms of tissue and cellular levels.

Measurement of IL-6 concentrations in septic patients receiving haemofiltration, showed a decrease with time with no clear increase in the ultrafiltrate because it is too big to be filtered by the membrane (Figure 5.2). However in contrast, IL-1β, which is a much smaller molecule is present in much higher concentrations in the filtrate than in serum, suggesting that

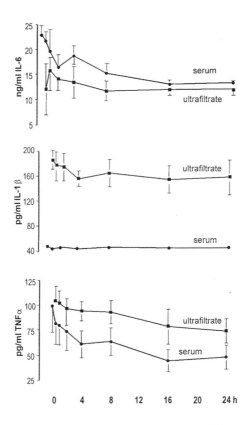

Figure 5.2   The effect of haemofiltration on serum and ultrafiltrate cytokine concentrations in patients with sepsis.

Table 5.2   Unresolved clinical questions

- Which type of membrane
- Length of therapy time
- Which patients
- Impact on outcome
- Adverse effects

IL-1β is filtered by the membrane. Serum concentrations of TNFα decrease in parallel with the ultrafiltrate concentration (Figure 5.2), suggesting that TNF is probably reduced by both adsorption and filtration although the size of the TNF molecule means that only around 15% is removed.

Summary

Systemic inflammation related to infection is common in the Intensive Care Unit. Infection, trauma and surgery initiates a pro-inflammatory response. This early phase can be followed by a post-aggressive immunodepression. Early organ failure may result from the non-tolerance of such inflammation processes. In this situation, it appears logical to modulate these reactions and allow the organs to tolerate inflammation. Vascular impairment with abnormal vascular permeability is frequent, thus amplifying interstitial oedema. Continuous haemofiltration may be beneficial although the mechanism on the inflammatory network remains to be clarified. However, studies have shown that haemofiltration reduces circulating endotoxin and low molecular weight mediators such as IL-1β, but not larger molecules such as TNFα and IL-6. It seems clear that continuous haemofiltration can remove excess water and solutes with a better tolerance than diuretics and/or intermittent haemodialysis. However there are no clinical data regarding the impact of haemofiltration on cell function and inflammatory phenotype.

Present development of haemofiltration is targeted to membrane pore size and adsorptive properties. However, before continuous haemofiltration can be recommended as a therapy rather than simply for renal support, multicentre trials focused on the impact of such therapy on organ dysfunction are required. There are certainly still many clinical questions which remain to be answered (Table 5.2).

References

1 Gotleib L, Barzilay E, Shustak A et al. Hemofiltration in septic ARDS. The artificial kidney as an artificial lung. Resuscitation 1986;**13**:123–32.
2 Barzilay E, Kessler D, Berlot G et al. Use of extracorporeal supportive techniques as additional treatment for septic induced multiple organ failure patients. Crit Care Med 1989;**17**:634–7.

3 Bellomo R, Tipping P, Boyce N. Continuous veno-venous hemofiltration with dialysis removes cytokines from the circulation of septic patients. *Crit Care Med* 1993;**21**:522–6.

4 Schiffl H, Lang SM, Konig A, Strasser T, Haider MC, Held E. Biocompatible membranes in acute renal failure: prospective case controlled study. *Lancet* 1994;**344**:570–2.

5 Natanson C, Esposito CJ, Banks SM. The sirens' songs of confirmatory sepsis trials: selection bias and sampling error. *Crit Care Med* 1998;**26**:1927–31.

6 Tetta C, Cavaillon JM, Schulze M *et al*. Removal of cytokines and activated complement components in an experimental model of continuous plasma filtration coupled with sorbent adsorption. *Nephrol Dial Transplant* 1998;**13**:1458–64.

7 Docke WD, Randow F, Syrbe U *et al*. Monocyte deactivation in septic patients: restoration by interferon gamma treatment. *Nature Med* 1997;**3**:678–81.

8 Losser MR, Bernard C, Beaudeux JL, Pison C, Payen D. Glucose modulates hemodynamic, metabolic, and inflammatory responses to lipopolysaccharide in rabbits. *J Applied Physiol* 1997;**83**:1566–74.

9 Meszaros K, Lang C, Bagby G, Spitzer J. *In vivo* glucose utilization by individual tissues during nonlethal hypermetabolic sepsis. *FASEB J* 1988;**2**:3083–6.

10 Journois D, Pouard P, Greeley WJ *et al*. Hemofiltration during cardiopulmonary bypass in pediatric cardiac surgery. *Anesthesiol* 1994;**81**:1181–9.

11 Journois D. Complement fragments and cytokines: production and removal as consequences of hemofiltration. *Contrib Nephrol* 1995;**116**:80–5.

12 Lee PA, Matson JR, Pryor RW, Hinshaw LB. Continuous arteriovenous hemofiltration therapy for staphylococcus aureus-induced septicemia in immature swine. *Crit Care Med* 1993;**21**:914–24.

13 Gomez A, Wang R, Unruh H *et al*. Hemofiltration reverses left ventricular dysfunction during sepsis in dogs. *Anesthesiol* 1990;**73**:671–85.

14 Grootendorst AF, van Bommel EF. The role of hemofiltration in the critically ill intensive care unit patient: present and future. *Blood Purif* 1993;**11**:209–23.

15 Mateo J, Cholley B, Teisseire B, Payen D. Endotoxin adsorption onto hemofiltration membranes improves hemodynamics in rabbit septic shock. *Am Rev Resp Dis* 1993;**147**:A98.

16 Mateo J, Bernard C, Teisseire L, Payen D. LPS adsorption prevents vascular depression during septic shock in rabbits. *Resp Crit Care Med* 1994;**149**:A657.

17 Di Scipio AW, Burchard KW. Continuous arteriovenous hemofiltration attenuates polymorphonuclear leukocyte phagocytosis in porcine intra-abdominal sepsis. *Am J Surg* 1997;**173**:174–80.

18 Aoki H, Kodama M, Tani T, Hanasawa K. Treatment of sepsis by extracorporeal elimination of endotoxin using polymyxin B-immobilized fiber. *Am J Surg* 1994;**167**:412–17.

19 Passaventi G, Buongiorno E, De-Fino G, Fuarola D, Coratelli P. The permeability of dialytic membranes to endotoxins: clinical and experimental findings. *Int J Artif Organs* 1989;**12**:505–8.

20 Cavaillon J, Munoz C, Fitting C, Misset B, Carlet J. Circulating cytokines: the tip of the iceberg? *Circ Shock* 1992;**38**:145–52.

6: Dopamine and dopexamine in the prevention of acute renal failure

ROBIN G WOOLFSON

Summary

Optimum renoprotection for patients at risk of developing renal failure remains elusive. This partly reflects the failure of most clinical studies to use reliable end-points to measure renal function and injury. Much interest has focused on dopamine but concerns about possible nephrotoxicity in diabetics and the adverse effects of α-adrenergic stimulation suggest that further studies are warranted. The development of other dopaminergic agents with improved pharmacological profiles, such as dopexamine, is very attractive. In patients undergoing major surgery, there are some data to suggest that dopexamine may be renoprotective but no studies using dopexamine to protect against radiocontrast media nephrotoxicity have been undertaken. The mortality and expense of patients who develop acute renal failure in hospital is high and the primary consideration has to be the development of effective renoprotection in these patients.

Introduction

Dopexamine is a dopaminergic agonist with β- but not α-adrenergic actions, whereas dopamine has unpredictable α-adrenergic actions, especially at higher doses. The renal actions of these two agents are therefore similar but the vasodilatory effects of dopexamine on the systemic and splanchnic circulations are preferable to those of dopamine. Most prospective studies which have investigated the potential renoprotective benefit of dopamine and dopexamine have involved patients undergoing either major cardiovascular surgery or radiocontrast media studies. This review will concentrate on the randomised controlled studies which have been undertaken in such patients, and attempt to clarify the evidence regarding the renoprotective roles of dopamine and dopexamine.

Hospital acquired renal dysfunction

Renal hypoperfusion and certain nephrotoxins such as radiocontrast media cause intrarenal vasoconstriction which may lead to parenchymal ischaemia and the development of acute tubular necrosis. Glomerular filtration rate (GFR) falls due to vasoconstriction, tubular obstruction by parenchymal oedema, desquamated epithelial cells and casts, and back-leak of glomerular filtrate through abnormally permeable tubular epithelia. The vulnerability of the tubular epithelium reflects its high metabolic activity and the physiological conditions of borderline hypoxia. Mismatch between energy supply and demand has been implicated in the pathogenesis of experimental acute tubular necrosis and this has formed the basis for clinical renoprotection.

There are few recent data regarding the epidemiology of hospital acquired acute renal failure. In a study from the United States, during 6 months in 1978–79, of 2200 consecutive admissions, the incidence of hospital acquired renal dysfunction in patients with normal or abnormal renal function was 5% of all admissions, with a mortality rate of 25%.[1] The causes of acute renal failure included post-operative hypovolaemia, congestive cardiac failure, radiocontrast injury and aminoglycoside therapy. Worryingly, 20% of these episodes of acute renal failure were drug induced and 55% were potentially avoidable episodes secondary to fluid and/or drug mismanagement. The mortality in patients who develop renal failure through hypoperfusion is much higher than that in, for example patients who receive an overdose of aminoglycosides. These results were supported by a second study from the USA which also showed substantially increased mortality in patients who developed acute renal failure following admission to hospital.[2]

Dopamine

Dopamine is a naturally occurring hormone which inhibits tubular Na/K-ATPase (responsible for the bulk of epithelial ATP consumption) and promotes vasodilatation, thereby increasing renal blood flow, glomerular filtration rate, natriuresis and diuresis. At low doses, dopaminergic actions prevail but as doses increase there is activation of β-adrenergic and then α-adrenergic receptors which leads to unpredictable increases in cardiac output, tachyarrhythmias, myocardial ischaemia and systemic vasoconstriction. Additional unwanted effects of dopamine include hypovolaemia

Table 6.1 Effects of dopamine

A.

Receptor	
Dose	Effect
1–2 µg/kg/min	dopaminergic agonist
3–10 µg/kg/min	β-adrenergic agonist
10–15 µg/kg/min	β- and α-adrenergic agonist
> 20 µg/kg/min	mostly α-adrenergic agonist

B.

Effects
Increased renal blood flow
Increased glomerular filtration rate
Natriuresis and diuresis
Afferent vasodilatation
Inhibition of Na/K-ATPase
Antagonises ADH

(due to excess diuresis), hypokalaemia, hypophosphataemia, respiratory depression and hyperprolactinaemia (Table 6.1). Randomised prospective controlled trials of the renoprotective role of dopamine have been restricted to two relatively homogenous pathological situations, namely following major surgery and radiocontrast media-induced injury.

Major surgery

Fifty-two patients undergoing elective coronary bypass received either dopamine or saline starting prior to and continuing for 24 hours after surgery.[3] Dopamine conferred no benefit in terms of improved serum creatinine or creatinine clearance in the post-operative period and had no significant effect on urine volume, although haemodynamic variables (cardiac index and systemic vascular resistance) were improved by dopamine in the immediate post-operative period. A later study of 37 patients undergoing major abdominal aortic surgery who received either dopamine or saline post-operatively for 24 hours found that dopamine increased urine output but had not improved renal function by day 5.[4] Haemodynamic monitoring was not undertaken but there was a non-significant increase in the incidence of myocardial infarction in dopamine recipients. This study therefore raised the concern that dopamine may be contraindicated in patients with significant ischaemic heart disease. Using sensitive measures of renal function and tubular injury, we have

37

recently studied 49 patients who underwent routine coronary artery bypass or single valve replacement for the first time and who were assigned to receive either dopamine or placebo from the induction of anaesthesia for a period of 48 hours.[5] All patients had normal renal function prior to surgery, with glomerular filtration (determined by isotope clearance) rates of approximately 75 ml/min. Glomerular filtration rates were not reduced at day 5 irrespective of whether patients received dopamine or placebo treatment. However, tubular epithelial injury as evidenced by albuminuria, urinary retinol binding protein, α-1-microglobulinuria and urinary NAG was reduced in dopamine recipients. These studies taken together suggest some degree of renoprotection from dopamine in patients undergoing major surgery.

Radiocontrast

Another clinical scenario in which pre-emptive renal protection may be beneficial is in patients undergoing radiocontrast interventions. In 60 patients with moderate pre-existing renal failure and serum creatinine concentrations of approximately 170 μmol/l, dopamine plus fluid resulted in a significant increase in creatinine clearance, compared to those who received fluids alone.[6] However, data from diabetics were not analysed separately in this study, which may be important given subsequent findings. Conversely, in a study of 222 patients who received radiocontrast media, dopamine did not appear to protect renal function more than placebo.[7] Fifty fluid resuscitated patients undergoing radiocontrast studies were assigned to receive a variety of vasodilators of which dopamine appeared to offer non-significant renoprotection to non-diabetics but was significantly nephrotoxic in diabetic patients.[8] Other studies have confirmed that optimum renoprotection against contrast nephropathy is best achieved with adequate pre-salination.[9,10] These studies taken together suggest that dopamine may be beneficial or at least harmless in non-diabetic patients at risk of radiocontrast nephropathy but may be harmful in those patients with diabetes.

Established acute renal failure

Dopamine has also been used in patients with established acute renal failure. In an early study from Thailand, 23 patients with falciparum malaria and acute renal failure, all of whom were treated with saline-loading and quinine, were studied.[11] Patients were divided into those with severe (creatinine 400 μmol/l) or very severe (creatinine 600 μmol/l) renal dysfunction and received treatment with furosemide plus or minus dopamine. In those patients with very severe injury, renal function worsened independent of treatment group but in the patients with less severe renal failure, the need for dialysis was avoided only if the furosemide plus dopamine combination therapy was prescribed. However, in a recent study of low ($<$ 3 μg/kg/min) or high ($>$ 3 μg/kg/min) dose dopamine versus placebo in 256 ICU patients, there was no difference in risk of death or the requirement for dialysis, regardless of dopamine dose.[12] We can therefore conclude that there are no significant data to support the routine use of dopamine therapy in patients with established acute renal failure.

Dopexamine

Dopexamine is a potent β_2-adrenergic and dopaminergic agonist (like dopamine), but without significant α-adrenergic activity (unlike dopamine). Whereas dopamine increases mean arterial pressure and cardiac index as a result of increased stroke volume, dopexamine has little effect on mean arterial pressure and increases cardiac index by reduction of systemic vascular resistance. These haemodynamic effects are responsible for dopexamine's naturetic and diuretic actions; undesirable systemic side effects of dopexamine include tachycardia, nausea and vomiting (Table 6.2). Clinical studies of dopexamine have been conducted in either healthy volunteers or patients undergoing major surgery.

Volunteer studies

In a study of 6 volunteers who received incremental doses of dopamine, dobutamine or dopexamine over 2 hours, dopexamine caused a significantly greater rise in heart rate than either dobutamine or dopamine, whereas

Table 6.2   Effects of dopexamine

A.
Receptor
β-2-adrenergic agonist Dopaminergic agonist Indirect β-1-adrenergic agonist No adrenergic activity

B.
Effect
Increased renal blood flow Natriuresis and diuresis Splanchnic vasodilatation Indirect inotropic and chronotropic action

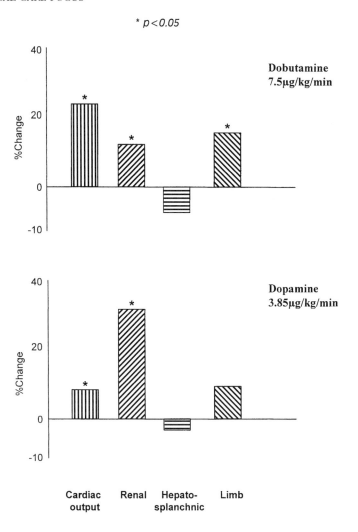

Figure 6.1 The relative changes in cardiac output and regional blood flow during maintenance infusions of dobutamine and dopamine in patients with moderately severe congestive heart failure (modified from Leier C et al., Am J Cardiol 1988; 62: 86E–93E with permission).

blood pressure was unchanged. Dopexamine did not increase renal plasma flow to the same extent as dopamine.[13] This lesser effect of dopexamine on renal blood flow was also demonstrated by Olsen *et al.*[14] who went on to show that only dopexamine increased glomerular filtration rate. These results reflect the differential effects of dopamine and dopexamine on systemic haemodynamics: dopamine increases cardiac output slightly but renal blood flow is increased markedly; and, dopexamine increases cardiac output markedly whilst renal blood flow is increased only slightly.

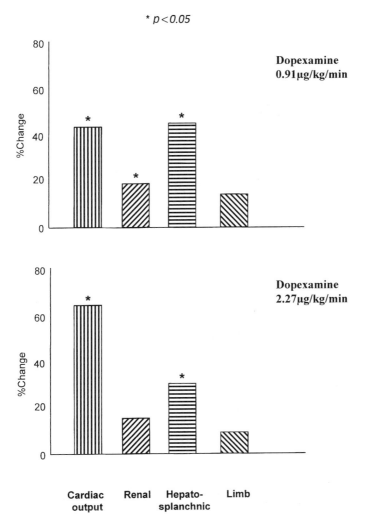

Figure 6.2   *The relative changes in cardiac output and regional blood flow in patients with congestive heart failure during two dose level infusions of dopexamine (modified from Leier C et al., Am J Cardiol 1988;* **62**: *86E–93E with permission).*

Major surgery

Twenty patients undergoing coronary artery bypass grafting received incremental doses of either dopexamine or dopamine immediately following induction of anaesthesia. In the patients who received dopexamine, cardiac index increased progressively and renal blood flow increased to a much lesser extent, whereas this pattern was reversed in dopamine-treated patients. The potential of dopexamine to protect renal function was

41

investigated in 32 patients undergoing infrarenal aortic surgery[15] in whom dopexamine or placebo infusion was begun pre-operatively and continued for 24 hours. Serum creatinine was lower in those patients receiving dopexamine than in the control group but creatinine clearances were not improved. Unfortunately this study did not include haemodynamic monitoring. A similar study of 44 patients undergoing coronary artery bypass grafting who received dopexamine at three different doses following induction of anaesthesia, found that there was a significant improvement in creatinine clearance, but this was unrelated to the concentration of drug received.[16] However, in a study of two matched groups of 12 patients undergoing orthotopic liver transplantation who were assigned to 48 hours of post-operative treatment with either dopexamine or dopamine, there was no difference in urine output or creatinine clearance between the two drugs, such that both appeared to be equally effective renoprotective agents.[17] A larger multicentre study comparing dopexamine and dopamine in patients with low cardiac output following cardiac surgery[18] found that urine output was maintained in both treatment groups but there were less cardiovascular events and better haemodynamics with dopexamine than dopamine. As a result, patients from the dopexamine group required concomitant vasodilatory support.

The systemic haemodynamic effects of dopexamine are more predictable and more beneficial than those of dopamine which is very relevant given the emerging concerns regarding the use of dopamine in patients at high risk of ischaemic heart disease. There are no clear data to suggest that the beneficial effects of dopexamine are due to intrarenal dopaminergic receptor activation and these more likely reflect increased cardiac output and systemic vasodilatation.

Conclusion

The theoretical renoprotective benefits of dopaminergic inhibition in patients exposed to renal hypoperfusion or nephrotoxicity remain attractive but many of the clinical studies of dopamine and dopexamine have been disappointingly inconclusive. In part, this reflects the failure to use precise measures of renal injury and the lack of adequate haemodynamic monitoring. Such deficiencies must be taken into account when designing future studies. Concerns regarding the adverse cardiac effects of dopamine in patients with ischaemic heart disease and the nephrotoxic effects of dopamine in patients with diabetic nephropathy exposed to radiocontrast underline the need to continue the search for better agents. Although preliminary studies have been very encouraging, the confirmation of a definite renoprotective role for dopexamine in patients undergoing major surgery requires further detailed studies. Similarly, the potential of dopexamine to reduce radiocontrast media-induced nephropathy deserves urgent exploration.

References

1 Hou SH, Bushinsky DA, Wish JB, Cohen JJ, Harrington JT. Hospital-acquired renal insufficiency: a prospective study. *Am J Med* 1983;**74**:243–8.

2 Shusterman N, Strom BL, Murray TG, Morrison G, West SL, Maislin G. Risk factors and outcome of hospital-acquired acute renal failure. Clinical epidemiologic study. *Am J Med* 1987;**83**:65–71.

3 Myles PS, Buckland MR, Schenk NJ, Cannon GB, Langley M, Davis BB, Weeks AM. Effect of "renal-dose" dopamine on renal function following cardiac surgery. *Anaesth Intensive Care* 1993;**21**:56–61.

4 Baldwin L, Henderson A, Hickman P. Effect of postoperative low-dose dopamine on renal function after elective major vascular surgery. *Ann Intern Med* 1994;**120**:744–7.

5 Sumeray M, Robertson C, Pugsley W, Bomanji J, Neild GH, Woolfson RG. Post-operative dopamine infusion is neither nephrotoxic nor renoprotective. *J Am Soc Nephrol* 1998;**9**:136A.

6 Hans B, Hans SS, Mittal VK, Khan TA, Patel N, Dahn MS. Renal functional response to dopamine during and after arteriography in patients with chronic renal insufficiency. *Radiology* 1990;**176**:651–4.

7 Hall KA, Wong RW, Hunter GC *et al*. Contrast-induced nephrotoxicity: the effects of vasodilator therapy. *J Surg Res* 1992;**53**:317–20.

8 Weisberg LS, Kurnik PB, Kurnik BR. Risk of radiocontrast nephropathy in patients with and without diabetes mellitus. *Kidney International* 1994;**45**:259–65.

9 Weinstein JM, Heyman S, Brezis M. Potential deleterious effect of furosemide in radiocontrast nephropathy. *Nephron* 1992;**62**:413–15.

10 Solomon R, Werner C, Mann D, D'Elia J, Silva P. Effects of saline, mannitol, and furosemide to prevent acute decreases in renal function induced by radiocontrast agents. *N Engl J Med* 1994;**331**:1416–20.

11 Lumlertgul D, Keoplung M, Sitprija V, Moollaor P, Suwangool P. Furosemide and dopamine in malarial acute renal failure. *Nephron* 1989;**52**:40–4.

12 Chertow GM, Sayegh MH, Allgren RL, Lazarus JM. Is the administration of dopamine associated with adverse or favorable outcomes in acute renal failure? Auriculin Anaritide Acute Renal Failure Study Group. *Am J Med* 1996;**101**:49–53.

13 Mousdale S, Clyburn PA, Mackie AM, Groves ND, Rosen M. Comparison of the effects of dopamine, dobutamine, and dopexamine upon renal blood flow: a study in normal healthy volunteers. *Br J Clin Pharmacol* 1988;**25**:555–60.

14 Olsen NV, Lund J, Jensen PF, Espersen K, Kanstrup IL, Plum I, Leyssac PP. Dopamine, dobutamine, and dopexamine. A comparison of renal effects in unanesthetized human volunteers. *Anesthesiol* 1993;**79**:685–94.

15 Welch M, Newstead CG, Smyth JV, Dodd PD, Walker MG. Evaluation of dopexamine hydrochloride as a renoprotective agent during aortic surgery. *Ann Vasc Surg* 1995;**9**:488–92.

16 Berendes E, Mollhoff T, Van Aken H *et al*. Effects of dopexamine on creatinine clearance, systemic inflammation, and splanchnic oxygenation in patients undergoing coronary artery bypass grafting. *Anesth Analg* 1997;**84**:950–7.

17 Gray PA, Bodenham AR, Park GR. A comparison of dopexamine and dopamine to prevent renal impairment in patients undergoing orthotopic liver transplantation. *Anaesthesia* 1991;**46**:638–41.

18 Rosseel PM, Santman FW, Bouter H, Dott CS. Postcardiac surgery low cardiac output syndrome: dopexamine or dopamine? *Intensive Care Medicine* 1997;**23**:962–8.

7: Furosemide and oxygen sparing

SAMUEL N HEYMAN

Introduction

Myocardial hibernation is a survival mechanism designed to maintain metabolic workload in the presence of local oxygen insufficiency. This review will focus on another illustration of the same concept, namely the renal medullary anginal syndrome, and the logic of a therapeutic approach in the clinical set-up of acute tubular necrosis, based on the inhibition of metabolic activity of renal tubular cells.

Renal oxygen delivery

About one-fifth of cardiac output is directed to the kidney, mainly for the filtration process, resulting in delivery of oxygen to the kidney in excess of 80 ml/min/100 g of tissue. This exceeds by far the oxygen supply to other vital organs such as the brain, myocardium and liver (Table 7.1). A very low fraction of delivered oxygen is extracted by the kidney, suggesting ample oxygen reserve in renal tissues. Paradoxically, however, the kidney is the organ which is most sensitive to hypoperfusion, with acute renal failure being one of the most frequent complications of hypotension. This paradox is related to a peculiar physiological gradient of intrarenal oxygenation, where the renal medulla functions at an ambient PO_2 as low as 20 mmHg.[1,2]

Intrarenal gradient of oxygenation

Physiological outer medullary hypoxia occurs as a result of both the medullary anatomy and high oxygen demand for reabsorption activity. Under normal physiological conditions the renal medulla functions at very low oxygen tensions. In studies using oxygen micro-electrodes,[3] a sharp decline in renal parenchymal oxygen tension was seen, from about 70 mmHg at the corticomedullary junction to approximately 20 mmHg in

45

Table 7.1   The renal medulla: life at the edge of anoxia

Organ		Oxygen delivery ml/min/100 g	Oxygen extraction %
Heart		17	65
Liver		12	18
Brain		11	34
Muscle		1	34
Kidney	total	84	10
	outer medulla	8	79

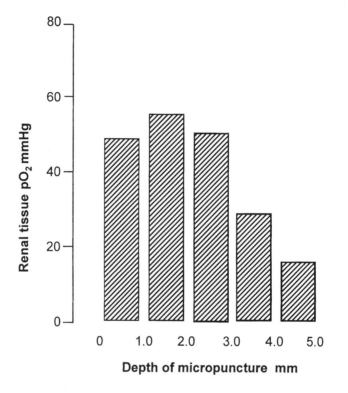

Figure 7.1   Mean renal tissue PO_2 measured under basal conditions at different depths of micropuncture into kidney parenchyma. Analysis of variance shows that PO_2 at 3–4 mm and 4–5 mm are significantly lower than at any of the superficial layers ($p < 0.0001$). Data are from kidneys in situ from 52 animals (reproduced with permission from Brezis M, Heyman SN, Dinour, D, Epstein FH, Rosen S. J Clin Invest 1991;**88**:390–5).

the outer medulla (Figure 7.1). Using rats, tissue PO_2 in the medulla is relatively consistent, although substantial variation in oxygen tension was found in the deep cortex, suggesting that low PO_2 probably exists in medullary rays as well.[3] The intrarenal gradient of oxygenation results from the peculiar anatomy of the medulla. The tubular segments at the level of the outer medulla are the straight portion of the proximal tubule, thin and thick ascending loops of Henlé and collecting ducts. These tubular segments generate the counter-current mechanism required for the process of urinary concentration and dilution. The regional vasculature originates from deep juxtamedullar nephrons that converge into vascular bundles – the vasa-recta. It runs down from cortical medullary rays and penetrates the medulla as far as the papillary tip. The capillary meshwork nourished from the vasa-recta supplies the interbundle zone and drains in part into ascending vasa-recta within the vascular bundles. The cross section illustrated in Figure 7.2 shows the architecture of the outer medulla with vascular bundles surrounded by tubules.[4]

A counter-current shunting of oxygen from descending to ascending vasa-recta exists so pre-capillary PO_2 markedly drops. As a result, in contrast to total renal oxygenation, medullary oxygen supply is quite limited at only 8 ml/min per 100 g of tissue. This limited oxygen supply is barely sufficient for the high oxygen consumption which is largely determined by reabsorptive work of thick ascending limbs. Thus outer medullary physiological hypoxia results from the combined effects of low regional oxygen delivery and high local oxygen consumption. The marginal oxygen reserve in the outer medulla is underscored by a very high oxygen extraction fraction – close to 80% – compared to the low total renal extraction fraction of only 10%. Continuous oxygen deprivation is reflected by the

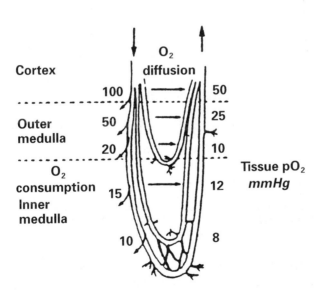

Figure 7.2   Diagram showing tissue PO_2 in different regions of the kidney in relation to oxygen diffusion and consumption (reproduced with permission from Brezis M, Rosen S, Silva P, et al. Renal ischemia: a new perspective. Kidney Internat. 1984;26:375–83).

high proportion of reduced cytochromes in the medulla in contrast to predominantly oxygenated forms in other tissues.

Medullary oxygen balance: lessons from the isolated perfused rat kidney

Studies in the isolated rat kidney clarify the importance of this physiological medullary hypoxia. In the model developed by Ross[5] the isolated kidney is mounted on a glass cannula inserted into the renal artery and continually perfused with circulating oxygenated perfusion medium. Urine is collected from the ureter and renal function is periodically monitored. At the conclusion of the experiment the kidney is perfusion-fixed for morphological examination. When isolated kidneys were perfused with erythrocyte-free oxygenated medium, hypoxic damage developed within 15 minutes, selectively affecting thick ascending limbs in the outer medulla.[6] Approximately 40% of thick limbs were injured following perfusion with erythrocyte-free medium, while anoxic perfusion resulted in extensive damage affecting some 95% of tubules. Severe necrotic lesions extended into medullary rays and included S3 segments as well, with deterioration of GFR and tubular function. When oxygen delivery was improved by the addition of haemoglobin or erythrocytes to the oxygenated medium, hypoxic damage was almost obliterated (Figure 7.3).[6]

Alterations in regional metabolic activity may also modulate a degree of outer medullary hypoxic injury. Reduction of oxygen consumption by the inhibition of ion transport activity of thick limbs with ouabain or with the loop diuretic furosemide attenuates hypoxic medullary damage.[6] Another way to diminish tubular absorption is to increase the oncotic pressure of the

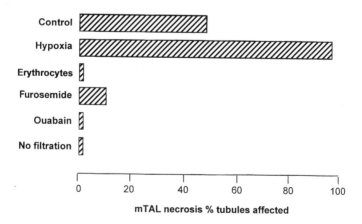

Figure 7.3   The percentage of injured tubules in isolated kidneys perfused with hypoxic medium and in the presence of erythrocytes, furosemide, ouabain or in the absence of filtration.[6]

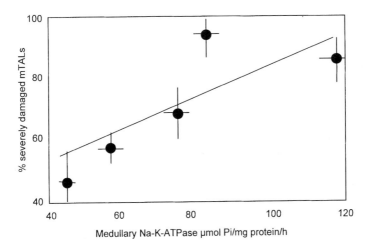

Figure 7.4   Relationship between NA-K-ATPase activity in outer medulla and the percentage of medullary thick ascending limb of loop of Henlé cells in the deepest portion of the outer medulla showing severe damage (reproduced with permission from Epstein FH, Silva P, Spokes K et al., Kidney Internat. *1989;36:768–72).*

perfusate by doubling the concentration of albumin. This leads to critical reduction of the glomerular filtration rate, while renal perfusion persists. In perfused but non-filtering kidneys, solute delivery to the distal nephron ceases and the metabolic activity of this region diminishes, again with the preservation of outer medullary hypoxic tubular damage.

In contrast enhanced metabolic activity increases outer medullary damage. In studies with the renal perfusion model, renal hypertrophy was induced by high protein diet or by prior contralateral nephrectomy or high potassium ingestion.[7] In these hypertrophic kidneys GFR is increased, tubular cells are larger with increased mitochondrial mass, and ion transporters work double shifts. There is a close correlation between sodium-potassium ATPase – a marker of tubular reabsorption activity – and hypoxic outer medullary damage. By contrast, in rats on low protein diet and low ATPase activity, damage is reduced (Figure 7.4). Thus under physiological conditions high outer medullary oxygen demand is hardly matched by sparse oxygen supply such that the outer medulla is susceptible to hypoxic injury during altered oxygen balance.

Renal protection mechanisms

With reference to the analogy of cardiac hibernation, renal anginal syndrome occurs, with the outer medulla functioning at the verge of anoxia (Table 7.2). Hypoxic injury may appear with decreased oxygen delivery or increased oxygen consumption. Oxygen sufficiency may be

Table 7.2   Outer medullary oxygen balance or the renal anginal syndrome

Oxygen sufficiency

- increased regional blood flow
- decreased regional metabolic activity

Oxygen insufficiency

- decreased regional blood flow
- increased regional metabolic activity

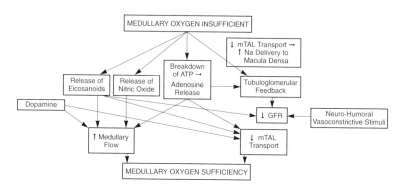

Figure 7.5   Schematic diagram of intrarenal oxygen balance. MTAL – medullary thick ascending limb of loop of Henlé; ATP – adenosine triphosphate; GRF – glomerular filtration rate (reproduced with permission from Heyman SN, Fuchs S, Brezis M. New Horizon 1995;3:597–607).

achieved by increasing oxygen delivery or with a reduction inhibition of thick limb metabolic activity. Even trivial daily changes in hydration state, dietary osmotic load, blood oxygenation or renal blood flow could alter the medullary oxygen balance. In order to protect the outer medulla from injury induced by oxygen imbalance, very efficient systems should operate to match oxygen delivery to requirement. Figure 7.5 summarises the complex physiological mechanisms which participate in the maintenance of medullary oxygen sufficiency.[2] These systems operate through both the control of regional blood flow and tubular solute reabsorption, which are the main determinants of regional oxygen consumption. Noteworthy, tubular absorption is determined to a large extent by the glomerular filtration rate, which in turn is in part governed by cortical blood flow. During effective volume depletion, characterised by increased neurohumoral vasoconstriction (increased sympathetic activity and the release of vasopressin and angiotensin II), GFR drops and solute delivery and hence transport activity through the distal nephron in this segment declines.

Unlike cortical blood flow, which is greatly influenced by the hydration state, outer medullary blood supply and oxygenation are largely preserved, or even increased, at various degrees of effective volume depletion, falling only during extreme renal hypoperfusion. For instance, the renal microcirculatory response to systemic hypotension induced by nitroprusside, is a fall in total and cortical renal blood flow and a paradoxical increase in medullary blood flow.[8] This cortical medullary redistribution of blood also occurs clinically during dehydration and hypovolaemia in low cardiac output states, cirrhosis and hypoalbuminaemia, allowing filtration predominantly in the deep juxtamedullary nephrons, thus optimising maximal urinary concentration. During systemic and cortical vasoconstriction, preservation of medullary flow is produced by the local paracrine action of vasodilating agents, including prostaglandins – in particular PGE_2 and prostacycline, adenosine, nitric oxide, dopamine and perhaps other yet unidentified mediators. Some of these agents also attenuate tubular metabolic work by decreasing GFR or by a direct inhibition of tubular reabsorption.

Where tubular damage develops, perhaps in response to extreme outer medullary oxygen imbalance with hypoxic tubular injury and increasing sodium delivery to the macula densa, defective tubular transport develops with consequent activation of the tubular glomerular feedback mechanism. As a result GFR then decreases leading to diminished tubular oxygen requirements with the restoration of oxygen sufficiency. Again some of these mediators previously mentioned, such as adenosine, participate in this phenomenon. The reduction in GFR during early renal failure should therefore be considered a protective mechanism for the preservation of medullary integrity, and preservation of medullary oxygenation. During systemic hypotension, although cortical flow and hence oxygenation falls, medullary oxygenation is not only maintained but may be substantially improved.

Medullary hypoxic damage

The physiological renal protective mechanisms described above are very effective and can compensate for each other. Thus, a single insult which alters medullary oxygen balance rarely causes acute renal impairment under either experimental conditions or in clinical practice. In contrast a combination of several insults or risk factors for medullary hypoxia are almost always present in patients with acute renal failure. For example, radiocontrast-induced nephropathy occurs almost exclusively in the presence of co-existing predisposing factors, and its incidence is proportional to their number.

A list of both experimental and clinical conditions for which a role for medullary hypoxic damage has been documented, is given in Table 7.3. The concept of medullary involvement in acute tubular necrosis stems from the first human morphologic evidence for distal tubular damage,

Table 7.3   Roles of medullary hypoxic damage in nephrotoxicity

- Non-steroidal anti-inflammatory agents
- Radiocontrast media
- Amphoteracin
- Cyclosporin
- Tacrolimus
- Myoglobin
- Ureteral obstruction
- Endotoxin

described in autopsies of World War II casualties with crush injuries and acute renal failure. The renal lesion was termed at that time as lower nephron nephrosis. The mechanism for renal damage in these patients was probably multifactorial including rhabdomyolysis, prolonged hypotension and sepsis.

We now know that the infusion of myoglobin in intact animals causes selective reduction in medullary blood flow[9] and a drop in medullary oxygenation associated with focal outer medullary hypoxic damage (Figure 7.6). These changes are often overlooked in the face of the profound proximal tubular nephrotoxic damage and tubular obstruction. Radiocontrast-mediated nephropathy is another example of acute renal failure with medullary hypoxic damage. Contrast administration is associated with a profound decline in renal parenchymal oxygenation which is most prominent at the outer medulla, reaching a PO_2 as low as 5–10 mmHg.[10] The mechanisms of contrast-induced medullary hypoxia are multiple and compound, with the final result of focal outer medullary hypoxic damage, amplified by co-existing circumstances which pre-dispose to medullary hypoxia.

Studies using rats have demonstrated the importance of pre-disposing risk factors in the development of radiocontrast injury. In animals pre-conditioned by chronic salt depletion and unilateral nephrectomy (to mimic effective volume depletion and reduced nephron mass respectively), frank selective outer medullary necrosis occurred, involving over a quarter of the medullary thick limb population.[10] The damage was mainly in those tubules most remote from vascular bundles, in contrast to tubules adjacent to vascular bundles, which were in general preserved.

The risk factors for contrast nephropathy are characterised by altered medullary oxygen balance or impaired defence mechanisms, designed to maintain medullary oxygenation.[11] For instance, effective volume depletion, hypotension, congestive failure, decompensated cirrhosis and nephritis are all characterised by excessive neurohumoral vasoconstrictive stimuli. Altered defensive mechanisms such as nitrovasodilatation occur in some of these conditions and may be particularly apparent in the elderly, and in patients with diabetes, atherosclerosis, hypotension and

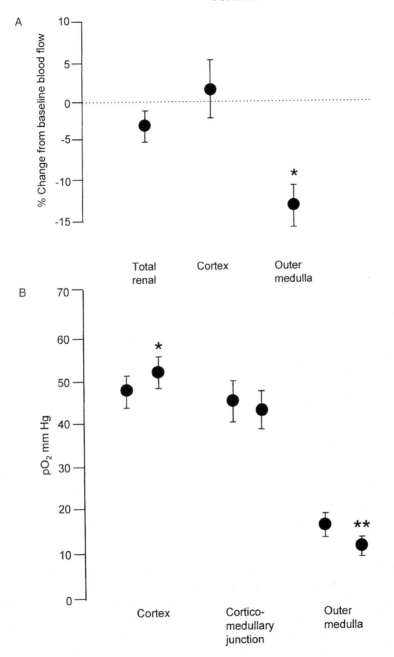

Figure 7.6   The effect of infusion of myoglobin in intact animals on (A) blood flow in areas of the rat kidney, and (B) the effect on oxygenation (reproduced from Heyman SN, Rosen S, Fuchs S, Epstein FH, Brezis M. J Am Soc Nephrol 1996;7:1066–74). $* = P < 0.05$; $** = P < 0.01$.

congestive failure. Co-administration of non-steroidal anti-inflammatory drugs (NSAIDs) markedly impairs medullary oxygenation through the inhibition of prostaglandin synthesis. Their use may be particularly dangerous during vasoconstrictive stimuli or defective nitrovasodilatation. Other nephrotoxic drugs such as cyclosporin or amphotericin may also compromise medullary blood flow.[2]

Acute renal failure: therapeutic approaches from the outer medullary point of view

Therapeutic strategies in the prevention or management of renal impairment should take medullary oxygen balance into account. The most important determinant for the prevention of renal failure is the identification of patients at risk and elimination of potential contributing factors. Unnecessary exposure to nephrotoxins or agents that may adversely effect medullary oxygen sufficiency, such as NSAIDs or radiocontrast agents should be avoided in this population. Correction of salt and volume depletion is paramount in the prevention of radiocontrast, amphotericin, cyclosporin and other nephrotoxic-hypoxic-mediated renal damage. Measures which stimulate intense glomeruli filtration in acute renal failure, such as the use of atrial natiuretic peptide analogues, theophylline, dopamine, or growth factors should be regarded with caution, since they all increase metabolic workload in the outer medulla and hence aggravate medullary hypoxia.[2]

Loop diuretics and medullary oxygenation

Loop diuretics block the active sodium-potassium-chloride co-transport in the apical membrane of thick limb tubular cells (Figure 7.7). However, the question of whether their use can improve medullary oxygenation and prevent or ameliorate the clinical syndrome of acute tubular necrosis is more complex.

In intact rats, furosemide abolishes the physiological outer medullary hypoxia.[8] This happens despite a marked fall in regional blood flow,[2,8,12] emphasising the role of reduced metabolic work and oxygen consumption rather than enhanced oxygen delivery as the cause of the improved medullary oxygenation. Furosemide also improved regional oxygenation in healthy volunteers, as shown by magnetic resonance imaging.[13] Furosemide also reverses medullary hypoxia produced by nephrotoxins. For instance, in rats given radiocontrast, medullary PO_2 declines substantially, is further intensified by the osmotic agent mannitol and is sharply normalised when furosemide is added.[8,14]

54

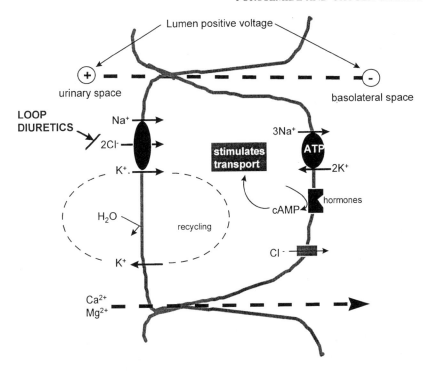

Figure 7.7   NaCl transport in the thick ascending limb and the site of action of loop diuretics.

Loop diuretics and prevention and amelioration of renal damage

Animal studies

The protective effect of furosemide in the isolated kidney is clear. A reduction of outer medullary damage of medullary thick ascending limbs and S3 segments is seen in furosemide or bumetanide-treated kidneys.[6,15] Since loop diuretics mainly work at the site of the thick ascending limb, why does furosemide protect the S3 segments? This can presumably be explained by the fact that as these segments are competing for limited oxygen supplies, decreasing the metabolic activity by medullary thick limbs increases the oxygen available for S3 segments.

The effect of loop diuretics on kidney function and integrity has also been examined *in vivo*. Rats subjected to chronic salt depletion and nephrectomy with resulting compensatory hypertrophy of the remaining kidney, were given radiocontrast medium and indomethacin. The rats developed acute renal failure and selective outer medullary hypoxic damage, affecting almost 30% of medullary thick limbs.[10] The administration of furosemide resulted

55

in almost complete prevention of tubular necrosis, although kidney function was only partially restored.[14] This may be explained by the large proportion of collapsed tubules, noted in the outer medulla, probably reflecting volume depletion. Fluid resuscitation with normal saline in addition to furosemide prevented tubular collapse and maintained renal function.

Clinical studies

Despite its protective effect in experimental settings the administration of loop diuretics has failed so far to prevent renal failure in clinical practice. Table 7.4 summarises the findings of four studies. Solomon *et al.*, in their well-controlled study, investigated the protective properties of diuretics in high risk patients undergoing radiocontrast studies. All these patients had some degree of pre-existing renal failure and they were all treated with intravenous fluid prior to the procedure. Both furosemide and mannitol aggravated renal failure whilst kidney function was maintained in the control group.[16] Similar conclusions can be drawn from another study of high risk patients with renal failure undergoing cardiac catheterisation, namely that renal function deteriorated in those patients treated with furosemide.[17] Both these studies stress the importance of pre-emptive hydration in high risk patients to prevent extensive tubular collapse. The second study illustrates that despite the rehydration protocol, furosemide induced volume depletion, perhaps explaining its negative impact in these studies.

Two other clinical studies also found no clinical advantage of furosemide prophylaxis. In a well-controlled report from Glasgow,[18] there was no benefit from furosemide in terms of renal function and overall survival in patients with established renal failure. In another report from Switzerland,[19]

Table 7.4   Clinical trials of prophylaxis with loop diuretics

Reference	Objective	Patients	Protocol	Results
14	prevention of contrast nephropathy	chronic renal failure	vigorous hydration ± bolus furosemide	deteriorating renal function
15	prevention of contrast nephropathy	chronic renal failure	vigorous hydration ± bolus furosemide	deteriorating renal function and negative fluid balance
16	impact on survival and kidney function	established acute renal failure	dopamine and mannitol ± repeated bolus furosemide or torasemide	no effect
17	prevention of ARF	major surgery	low dose furosemide infusion	no effect

Table 7.5   Issues to consider in trials of loop diuretics

- Inadequate rehydration
- Patient selection (low/high risk; prophylaxis; established renal failure)
- Other drugs (dopamine; mannitol)
- Method of administration (bolus or infusion)

patients undergoing major operations had similar slight reductions in kidney function with and without prophylactic treatment with furosemide. None of these patients consequently developed acute renal failure requiring dialysis. It should be noted that continuous low dose furosemide was given in this study compared to bolus administration (inducing medullary vasoconstriction) in previous studies.

Some of these disappointing results are further confused by lack of comparability between study design. These issues include the degree of fluid replacement in diuretic treated patients, the patient groups themselves, the administration of other drugs such as dopamine and mannitol, and the way in which the furosemide is administered (Table 7.5).

Summary

Low medullary oxygenation results from abundant oxygen requirement for tubular reabsorptive activity, hardly matched by a limited regional oxygen supply. Medullary oxygenation is strictly balanced by control mechanisms, designed to match regional oxygen supply and consumption, and their failure renders the outer medulla susceptible to acute or repeated episodes of hypoxic injury, leading to acute tubular necrosis, or chronic tubulo-interstitial changes, respectively.

Interventions to enhance regional blood supply and decrease local tubular reabsorption seem to be a logical approach for the prevention of outer medullary oxygen insufficiency and hypoxic injury. Paradoxically, most therapeutic interventions (such as theophylline, mannitol or atrial natiuretic peptide analogues) result in increased glomerular filtration and tubular oxygen consumption, and may enhance tubular hypoxic damage.[20] Selective cortical vasoconstriction and decline in glomerular filtration rate during renal hypoperfusion or acute tubular necrosis are protective measures, decreasing reabsorption workload and preserving tubular integrity.

The loop diuretic furosemide improves medullary oxygenation by inhibition of solute reabsorption and oxygen requirement and improves hypoxic damage in animal models of renal injury. However, loop diuretics failed to ameliorate established renal failure or prevent post-operative decline in renal function in clinical practice. Moreover, radiocontrast induced nephropathy in high risk patients was worsened by furosemide. In conclusion, there is no evidence that loop diuretics may ameliorate or prevent acute tubular necrosis and additional experimental and clinical studies are required to address their potential protective properties.

References

1 Brezis M, Rosen S. Mechanisms of disease: hypoxia of the renal medulla: implications for disease. *N Engl J Med* 1995;**332**:647–55.

2 Heyman SN, Fuchs S, Brezis M. The role of medullary ischemia in acute renal failure. *New Horizons* 1995;**3**:597–607.

3 Brezis M, Heyman SN, Dinour D, Epstein FH, Rosen S. Role of nitric oxide in renal medullary oxygen balance. Studies in isolated and intact rat kidneys. *J Clin Invest* 1991;**88**:390–5.

4 Brezis M, Rosen S, Silva P *et al.* Renal ischemia: a new perspective. *Kidney Internat* 1984;**26**:375–83.

5 Ross BD, Epstein FH, Leaf A. Sodium reabsorption in the perfused rat kidney. *Am J Physiol* 1973;**225**:1165–71.

6 Brezis M, Rosen S, Silva P *et al.* Transport activity modifies thick ascending limb damage in the isolated perfused kidney. *Kidney Internat* 1984;**25**:65–72.

7 Epstein FH, Silva P, Spokes K *et al.* Renal medullary Na-K-ATPase and hypoxic injury in perfused rat kidneys. *Kidney Internat* 1989;**36**:768–72.

8 Brezis M, Agmon Y, Epstein FH. Determinants of intrarenal oxygenation I. Effects of diuretics. *Am J Physiol* 1994;**267**: F1059–62.

9 Heyman SN, Rosen S, Fuchs S, Epstein FH, Brezis M. Myoglobinuric acute renal failure in the rat: A role for medullary hypoperfusion, hypoxia and tubular obstruction. *J Am Soc Nephrol* 1996;**7**:1066–74.

10 Heyman SN, Brezis M, Epstein FH, Spokes K, Silva P, Rosen S. Early renal medullary hypoxic injury from radiocontrast and indomethacin. *Kidney Internat* 1991;**40**:632–42.

11 Heyman SN, Rosen S, Brezis M. Radiocontrast nephropathy: A paradigm for the synergism between toxic and hypoxic insults in the kidney. *Exp Nephrol* 1994;**2**:153–7.

12 Heyman SN, Karmeli F, Rachmilewitz D, Haj Yehia A, Brezis M. Intrarenal nitric oxide monitoring with a clark-type electrode: potential pitfalls. *Kidney Internat* 1997;**51**:1619–23.

13 Prasad PU, Edelman RR, Epstein FH. Noninvasive evaluation of intrarenal oxygenation with BOLD MRI. *Circulation* 1996;**94**:3271–5.

14 Heyman SN, Brezis M, Greenfield Z, Rosen S. Protective role of furosemide and saline in radiocontrast-induced renal failure in the rat. *Am J Kidney Dis* 1989;**14**:377–85.

15 Heyman SN, Rosen S, Epstein FH, Spokes K, Brezis M. Loop diuretics reduce hypoxic damage to proximal tubules of the isolated perfused kidney. *Kidney Internat* 1994;**45**:981–5.

16 Solomon R, Werner C, Mann D *et al.* Effects of saline, mannitol and furosemide on acute decreases in renal function induced by radiocontrast agents. *N Engl J Med* 1994;**331**:1416–20.

17 Weinstein JM, Heyman SN, Brezis M. Potential deleterious effect of furosemide in radiocontrast nephropathy. *Nephron* 1992;**62**:413–15.

18 Shilliday IR, Quinn JK, Allison ME. Loop diuretics in the management of acute renal failure: a prospective, double blind, placebo controlled, randomized study. *Nephrol Dial Transplant* 1997;**12**:2592–6.

19 Hager B, Betschart M, Krapf R. Effect of postoperative intravenous loop diuretics on renal function after major surgery. *Schweiz Med Wochenschr* 1996;**126**:666–73.

20 Heyman SN, Rosen S, Brezis M. The renal medulla: Life at the edge of anoxia. *Blood Purif* 1997;**15**:232–42.

8:   Experimental drugs to prevent renal failure

ADRIAN J VOETS

Introduction

For the purpose of this review acute renal failure (ARF) is defined as a rapid, abrupt deterioration in intrinsic renal function, excluding pre-renal and post-renal causes, apart from glomerular nephritis and interstitial – or acute tubular – nephritis. ARF is a prevalent disorder in patients on the Intensive Care Unit, with an incidence, depending on population, of up to 15%.[1] Established ARF in the critically ill is associated with increased morbidity, increased length of stay and increased costs, and carries a mortality rate of about 65%.[2] Despite considerable effort, the mortality rate has not declined in the last decade, probably due to the increasing age and co-morbidity of the Intensive Care Unit population.[3] Any management strategy, therefore, which prevents or reduces the incidence and morbidity of acute renal failure will be of benefit. This review will concentrate on clinical studies and discuss the problems involved with such studies.

Problems

Assessing renal function

Under stable conditions the measurement of serum creatinine concentration and creatinine clearance is a useful means of assessing glomerular filtration rate i.e. renal function. However, when patients may be unstable such as after major surgery, renal function becomes much more difficult to accurately measure. In a survey of tests of renal function,[4] it was concluded that serial measurement of creatinine clearance was the single most sensitive parameter, but clearly this is extremely labour intensive. In reality, serum creatinine is being used clinically to diagnose renal failure. Serum creatinine increases only when 50% of renal function is lost – resulting in a significant delay in diagnosing ARF – and is also influenced by non-renal factors.

60

Defining acute renal failure

Although it appears that renal failure is easily defined, Novis *et al.*, 1994, showed that of 28 studies, involving over 10 000 patients, no two studies used the same criteria to define renal failure,[2] such that comparison of data remains very difficult and meta-analysis impossible. It is easy to see how studies of preventative therapy need intricate planning to succeed.

Extrapolating animal studies

Although studies in animals provide vital insight into mechanisms of renal disease and are essential to our understanding, no experimental model accurately reflects physiological and pathological changes in man. In addition, inter-species differences may cause problems. This is illustrated well by the difference in distribution of endothelin receptors in different species.[5] The extrapolation of results from animal studies to man is therefore fraught with problems.

Clinical setting

The clinical characteristics or setting of patient studies are important. Often patients with differing disease characteristics are grouped together causing the problem of "case mix". However, the original insult causing renal failure has profound implications for both the manifestations and course of renal dysfunction. In addition, patients may be grouped at various time points in disease evolution as "early" or "late" – the latter carrying a worse prognosis – and independently of disease severity. The pathogenesis of renal dysfunction, for example ischaemic or nephrotoxic, is important too, since nephrotoxic renal failure seems to confer a better prognosis, although acute renal failure may often be multi-factorial. An example of this is provided by aminoglycoside toxicity, where both nephrotoxic and ischaemic mechanisms are involved. An example of this is provided by the use of aminoglycosides in sepsis, where both nephrotoxic and ischaemic mechanisms are involved.

Urine output is also crucial, since patients with oliguria frequently have a worse course than those who continue to pass urine, presumably representing greater renal damage. Co-morbidity must also be considered, and can be easily quantified using the APACHE score. Although renal function has an effect on mortality,[6,7] co-morbidity is probably more important. It is generally considered that patients die *with* renal failure and not *from* it.[8] It is therefore clear that in clinical studies, these factors which have such marked influence on course, prognosis and outcome should be realised and considered.

Timing of interventions

Of paramount importance is the timing of any intervention. Strictly speaking, prevention or prophylaxis means intervening before the insult which leads to renal dysfunction, although clearly this is not always practical. Treatment, on the other hand, means intervention after renal dysfunction is apparent, and this is often arbitrarily defined as the first 48 hours, or estabilished phase of ARF.

Defining end-points

Clearly the definition of both the goals of treatment and clinical end-points is difficult. Serum creatinine concentrations or creatinine clearance are often used; for example a rise of 50% above baseline levels and patterns in the change in creatinine clearance may be useful as an end-point. As a goal of therapy, these measures may be less suitable and it is hard to understand the clinical relevance of a transient change in serum creatinine. Blood urea nitrogen is dependent not only on renal function, but also on non-renal factors. It is a subjective measure, but as an indicator of a requirement for dialysis, along with uncontrollable hyperkalaemia, acidosis and fluid overload, it may be a useful treatment goal as well as an end-point of a study. Urine output alone is not a reliable end-point, although recovering urine output in a previously oliguric patient may be useful.[9,10]

As an easily defined marker, mortality is well suited as a goal of treatment. However, as previously mentioned, mortality is heavily influenced by co-morbidity. Common causes of death are sepsis, cardiovascular abnormalities and pulmonary dysfunction, and of course withdrawal of life support measures.[1] Mortality is therefore non-specific and hence not appropriate as an end-point of clinical studies.

Drugs in acute renal failure

A large number of different drugs (Table 8.1), including vasoactive agents, free radical scavengers and others have all been used in experimental animal models of renal failure.[4] In addition, a list half as long has been used clinically (Table 8.2). These drugs address well defined pathophysiological mechanisms, including vasoconstriction, desquamation of tubular cells, tubular obstruction and transtubular back-leak.[11] Vasoactive agents attempt to increase renal blood flow (e.g. low dose dopamine and atrial natriuretic factor); diuretics increase urine flow and hence reduce tubular obstruction. Some compounds act on more than one mechanism at once, such as mannitol, which reduces tubular obstruction by reducing epithelial swelling, and also acts as an antioxidant. Loop diuretics such as furosemide lower epithelial ATP and oxygen requirements by inhibiting ion transport in addition to their diuretic effects. To date no drug has been shown to be consistently beneficial.[12]

Since vasoconstriction has a pivotal rule in the pathophysiology of ARF, clinical studies with vasoactive drugs are likely to be most promising. The

Table 8.1   Drugs used in experimental acute renal failure

Vasoactive agents
  propranolol
  phenoxybenzamine
  clonidine
  bradykinin
  acetylcholine
  prostaglandin E1
  prostaglandin E2
  prostacyclin
  saralasin
  captopril
  verapamil
  nifedipine
  nitrendipine
  diltiazem
  chlorpromazine
  atrial natriuretic peptide
  theophylline
  antiendothelin antibody
  dopamine
	Neutrophil depletion or inhibition of leucocyte
	adhesion
	  antineutrophil serum
	  nitrogen mustard
	  anti-CD 18 antibody
	  anti-ICAM-1 antibody
	
	Elastase cathepsin inhibitors
	  elgin C
	
	Agents to restore cell energetics
	  ATP-MgCl$_2$
	  thyroxin
	  glycine
	
	Anticoagulants and antiplatelet agents
	  pentoxyfylline
	  pipyridamole
	  heparin
	  aspirin

Diuretics
  mannitol
  furosemide
	Growth factors
	  epidermal growth factors
	  insulin-like growth factor-1

Inhibitors or scavengers of free radicals
  allopurinol
  oxypurinol
  deferoxamine
  dimethylthiourea
  dimethylsulfoxide
  superoxide dismutase
  catalase
  glutathione
  probucol
  diethylthiocarbamate
	Inhibitors of cast formation
	  RGD peptides
	
	Alkalinising agents
	  tri(hydroxymethyl)methane

Table 8.2   Drugs used in clinical acute renal failure

Vasoactive agents
  dopamine
  phenoxybenzamine
  phentolamine
  prostaglandin A1
  prostaglandin E1
  verapamil
  diltiazem
  nifedipine
  atrial natriuretic peptide
	Toxin chelators, scavengers, or inhibitors
	  dimercaprol
	  edetate calcium disodium
	  penicillamine
	  N-acetylcysteine
	  leukovorin
	  allopurinol
	  haptoglobin
	  sodium thiosulfate
	  ethanol
	  4-methylpyrazole

Diuretics
  mannitol
  furosemide
  ethacrynic acid
	Alkalising agents
	  Sodium bicarbonate

review will now present some of those critical studies, but the results should be considered in the light of the problems discussed above.

Atrial natriuretic peptide

Atrial natriuretic peptide (ANP) is produced as a pro-protein, which, after proteolytic cleavage yields the 28 amino acid mature ANP product. There are two other types of natriuretic peptide; brain type (BNP) and C type (CNP), source unknown. ANP is produced mainly in cardiac atria, but also occurs in the kidney, where it is called urodilatin. The strongest stimulus for ANP release is increased tension of the atrial wall, through increased venous return to the heart. Endothelin, vasopressin and catecholamines also directly stimulate ANP release. The effect of ANP is mediated through its interaction with one of three receptors, and the half life in plasma is around 5 minutes.[13] The actions of ANP are summarised in Table 8.3.

ANP causes vasodilatation, increases venous capacitance and raises haematocrit through increased permeability. Within the kidney, ANP raises glomerular filtration rate, lowers renin production and causes natriuresis and diuresis. Aldosterone production in the adrenals decreases. Within the central nervous system, sympathetic outflow and neuroendocrine function is lowered through decreased corticotrophin levels. Water intake and salt appetite is decreased. These actions lead to decreased blood pressure and lower venous volume, completing the feedback loop. In many ways ANP it could be considered to have an action like that of "endogenous furosemide".

ANP has been administered both prophylactically and as treatment for ARF. Earlier this year a prospective, randomised control study was published which described the use of ANP in the prevention of radiocontrast

Table 8.3   Actions of atrial natriuretic peptide

- Cardiovascular
    vasodilatation
    increases venous capacitance
    increases permeability

- Renal
    increases GFR
    increases $U_{Na}V$
    increases UV
    decreases renin

- Adrenal
    decreases aldosterone

- Central nervous system
    decreases sympathetic outflow
    decreases neuroendocrine function
    decreases corticotropin
    decreases salt appetite
    decreases water intake

induced nephropathy.[14] The study included 247 patients with chronic renal dysfunction, which was defined as serum creatinine above 132 μmol/l. All patients were well hydrated and were randomised to receive either anaritide, a synthetic analogue of ANP, at one of three doses, or placebo. Radiocontrast nephropathy was defined as either an absolute increase in serum creatinine of 44 μmol/l or a relative increase of 25% above baseline. The incidence of nephropathy was similar in all four groups, at approximately 23%. It was concluded that ANP prophylaxis did not reduce the incidence of radiocontrast-induced nephropathy in patients with pre-existing chronic renal failure. These rather disappointing results confirmed those of a previous smaller preventative study in which anaritide failed to prevent ARF following cadaveric renal transplant.[15]

In the treatment of established ARF, very encouraging results were obtained initially in a small single centre study using anaritide.[16] This prompted a larger randomised controlled study of ANP treatment in 504 patients with acute tubular necrosis.[9] The inclusion criteria were acute tubular necrosis with an increase in creatinine of 88 μmol/l in 48 hours despite optimal fluid status. Patients who had received previous dialysis, who had chronic renal insufficiency, previous renal transplantation or low systolic blood pressure were excluded. The administration of diuretics and dopamine was allowed, at the discretion of the physician. The primary end-point was dialysis-free survival at 21 days and dialysis requirement at day 14. Secondary end-points were mortality from any cause and change in serum creatinine at day 21. There was no difference between patients receiving placebo and those receiving ANP, based on any end-point. However, a prospectively defined sub-group based on urinary output showed that ANP significantly increased dialysis-free survival and reduced the need for dialysis. In the non-oliguric group dialysis-free survival was decreased, however. It was concluded therefore that there is no benefit of ANP treatment in patients with acute tubular necrosis but it may improve dialysis-free survival in patients with oliguria. ANP may be detrimental in those without oliguria, probably through an increased incidence of hypotensive episodes. In summary, ANP may not be the way forward in preventing or treating acute renal failure.

Endothelin receptor antagonist

Another very promising compound is endothelium receptor antagonist. Endothelin was originally isolated from vascular endothelial cells. It is produced as pre-pro-endothelin, which is cleaved to form "big endothelin" and finally, through the action of endothelin converting enzyme, to the 21 amino acid endothelin. There are three known isoforms of endothelin, endothelins 1, 2 and 3. Endothelin 1 (ET1), our main substance of interest, is produced mainly by endothelial and smooth muscle cells, in response to hypoxia and shear stress. Endothelin 2 (ET2) occurs mainly in the

Table 8.4   Actions of endothelin

- Cellular
    increases cytosolic calcium concentration from
        (i) intracellular stores and
        (ii) extracellular calcium after recruitment of calcium channels

- Biological
    long-lasting vasoconstriction, mediated by calcium
    release of ANP in right atrium
    mitogenic function vascular smooth muscle cells
    release of pituitary hormones
    renal sodium retention

---

kidney and the intestines and the source of endothelium 3 (ET3) is as yet unknown.[17] The actions of endothelin are summarised in Table 8.4.

ET1 diffuses from the abluminal side to receptors on nearby cells in the interstitium and only a very small amount arrives in the vascular lumen. It acts therefore predominantly in a paracrine fashion. The endothelins activate receptors located on the cell membrane. There are two types of receptors, type A, and type B. Type A receptors are located on the vascular smooth muscle cells and in the right atrium and have high affinity for ET1. Type B receptors are primarily located on endothelial cells and have equal affinity for ET1 and ET3. In the kidney receptors have been demonstrated in the inner medulla, the vasa-recta, the mesangium and the glomeruli. Type A receptors are mainly involved in endothelin-mediated venal vasoconstriction.

Following receptor coupling, endothelin increases intracellular calcium through release from intracellular stores, and by mobilising extracellular calcium after recruitment of calcium channels. Of course here lies the rationale the use of calcium channel blockers in acute renal failure. The long lasting vasoconstricting effects of endothelin are attributed to increased intracellular calcium. Other biological assets are the release of atrial natriuretic peptide in the right atrium, and as a growth factor, endothelin promotes proliferation of smooth muscle cells, and regulates pituitary hormone release. In the kidney it causes sodium retention.

Endothelin has been implicated in the pathogenesis of a number of cardiovascular and renal diseases (Table 8.5). However, this is based largely on the finding that endothelin concentrations have been found to be elevated, and it is unclear whether this represents increased production or decreased clearance.[18]

In acute renal failure, endothelin is thought to be responsible for the long lasting vasoconstriction of the vas afferens, causing a disproportionate decrease in glomerular filtration rate compared to renal blood flow. This was proposed shortly after its discovery in 1988, based on the time-effect relationship of plasma levels of endothelin and signs of ARF.[19] The causative role of endothelin has been studied using both endothelin

Table 8.5   Pathological roles of endothelin

- Cardiovascular
    acute myocardial infarction
    congestive heart failure
    generalised atherosclerosis
    essential hypertension
    cerebral vasospasm in subarachnoid haemorrhage
    primary pulmonary hypertension

- Renal
    chronic renal failure
    cyclosporin-A induced nephrotoxicity
    radiocontrast-induced nephropathy
    hepatorenal syndrome
    (post-ischaemic) acute renal failure

receptor antagonists and calcium channel blocking agents. In various animal models of acute renal failure marked improvements in renal function were shown following endothelin receptor antagonist therapy as a preventive measure.[18] However, there have been no clinical studies to date on its use in acute renal failure, although there has been a recent study of an oral non-peptide endothelin receptor antagonist, bosentan, in patients with essential hypertension.[20] This may suggest, however, that the hypotensive effect of endothelin receptor antagonists may be a disadvantage in acute renal disease. Clearly further research will have to delineate the exact role of such agents in clinical ARF.

Calcium channel blockers have proven to counteract the renal effects of endothelin in volunteers,[21,22] supporting the role of ET-1 in ARF. In malaria induced nephropathy[23] renal transplantation and cyclosporin induced nephropathy[24,25] small but in significant differences were found, whereas in radiocontrast nephropathy no difference in renal function regardless of calcium channel blocker therapy was shown.[26]

Other new therapies for the future might include growth factors such as epidermal, hepatocyte or insulin-like growth factor,[27] which should hasten tubular recovery, anti-ICAM antibodies interfering with the adhesion of neutrophils and disintegrins counteracting tubular obstruction.[10]

Conclusion

To date, no drug has been shown to be of benefit in preventing or treating ARF. It is my opinion that endothelin receptor antagonist may have a future role in the prevention and therapy of acute renal failure, possibly in combination with growth factors. However, it is clear that there is still a great need for properly conducted randomised controlled trials, with clearly defined criteria to define renal dysfunction, and perhaps more importantly, well defined patient groups, to address the problems of co-morbidity, age etc. Such trials will help to produce evidence based guidelines for the prevention of acute renal failure.

References

1. Thadhani R, Pascual M, Bonventre JV. Acute renal failure. *N Engl J Med* 1996;**334**:1448–60.
2. Novis BK, Roizen MF, Aronson S, Thisted RA. Association of preoperative risk factors with postoperative acute renal failure. *Anesth Analg* 1994;**78**:143–9.
3. Tumev JH. Why is mortality persistently high in acute renal failure? *Lancet* 1990;**335**:971.
4. Kellen M, Aronson S, Roizen MF, Barnard J, Thisted RA. Predictive and diagnostic tests of renal failure: a review. *Anesth Analg* 1994;**78**:134–42.
5. Nambi P. Endothelin receptors in normal and diseased kidneys. *Clin Exp Pharm Physiol* 1996;**23**:326–30.
6. Levy EM, Viscoli CM, Horwitz RI. The effect of acute renal failure on mortality. A cohort analysis. *JAMA* 1996;**275**:1489–94.
7. Chertow GM, Levy EM, Hammermeister KE, Grover F, Dalev J. Independent association between acute renal failure and mortality following cardiac surgery. *Am J Med* 1998;**104**:343–8.
8. Prough DS. Still lethal after all these years. *Crit Care Med* 1996;**24**:189–90.
9. Allgren RL, Marbury TC, Rahman SN *et al*. Anaritide in acute tubular necrosis. *N Engl J Med* 1997;**336**:8288–94.
10. Alkhunaizi AM, Schrier RW. Management of acute renal failure: new perspectives. *Am J Kidney Dis* 1996;**28**:315–28.
11. Bonventre JV. Mechanisms of ischemic acute renal failure. *Kidney International* 1993;**43**:1160–78.
12. Conger JD. Drug therapy in acute renal failure. In: Lazarus JM, Brenner BM (eds.) Acute renal failure 3rd ed. Churchill Livingstone, New York, 1993.
13. Levin ER, Gardner DG, Samson WK. Natriuretic peptides. *N Engl J Med* 1998;**339**:321–8.
14. Kurnik BR, Allgren RL, Genter FC, Solomon RJ, Bates ER, Weisberg LS. Prospective study of atrial natriuretic peptide for the prevention of radiocontrast-induced nephropathy. *Am J Kidney Dis* 1998;**31**:674–80.
15. Sands JM, Neylan JF, Olson RA, *et al*. Atrial natriuretic factor does not improve the outcome of cadaveric renal transplantation. *J Am Soc Nephrol* 1991;**1**:1081–6.
16. Rahman SN, Kim GE, Mathew AS, *et al*. Effects of atrial natriuretic peptide in clinical acute renal failure. *Kidney Int* 1994;**45**:1731–8.
17. Levin ER. Endothelins. *N Engl J Med* 1995;**333**:356–63.
18. Kohan DE. Endothelin in the normal and diseased kidney. *Am J Kidney Dis* 1997;**29**:2–26.
19. Firth JD, Ratcliffe PJ, Raine AE, Ledingham JGG. Endothelin: an important factor in acute renal failure? *Lancet* 1988;**332**:1179–82.
20. Krum H, Viskoper RJ, Lacourciere Y, *et al*. The effect of an endothelin receptor antagonist bosentan on blood pressure in patients with essential hypertension. *N Engl J Med* 1998;**338**:784–90.
21. Kiowski W, Lüscher TF, Linder L, Bühler FR. Endothelin-1-induced vasoconstriction in humans. Reversal by calcium channel blockade but not by nitrovasodilators or endothelium-derived relaxing factor. *Circulation* 1991;**83**:469–75.

22. Rabelink TJ, Kaasjager KAH, Boer P, Stroes EG, Braam B, Koomans HA. Effects of endothelin-1 on renal function in humans: implications for physiology and pathophysiology. *Kidney Int* 1994;**46**:376–81.
23. Lumertgul D, Wongmekiat O, Sirivanichai C, *et al.* Intrarenal infusion of gallopamil in acute renal failure. A preliminary report. *Drugs* 1991;**42**(suppl 1):44–50.
24. Neumayer HH, Wagner K. Prevention of delayed graft function in cadaver kidney transplants by diltiazem: outcome of two prospective randomized clinical trials. *J Cardiovasc Pharmacol* 1987;**10**(suppl 10):S170–177.
25. Frei U, Harms A, Bakovic-Alt R, Pichlmayr R, Koch KM. Calcium channel blockers for kidney protection. *J Cardiovasc Pharmacol* 1990;**16**(suppl 6):S11–15.
26. Cacoub P, Baumelou A, Jacbs C. No evidence for protective effects of nifedipine against radio-contrast-induced acute renal failure. *Clin Nephrol* 1988;**29**:215–20.
27. Hammerman MR, Miller SB. Therapeutic use of growth factors in renal failure. *J Am Soc Nephrol* 1994;**5**:1–11.